Vintage Hair Styles of the 1940s

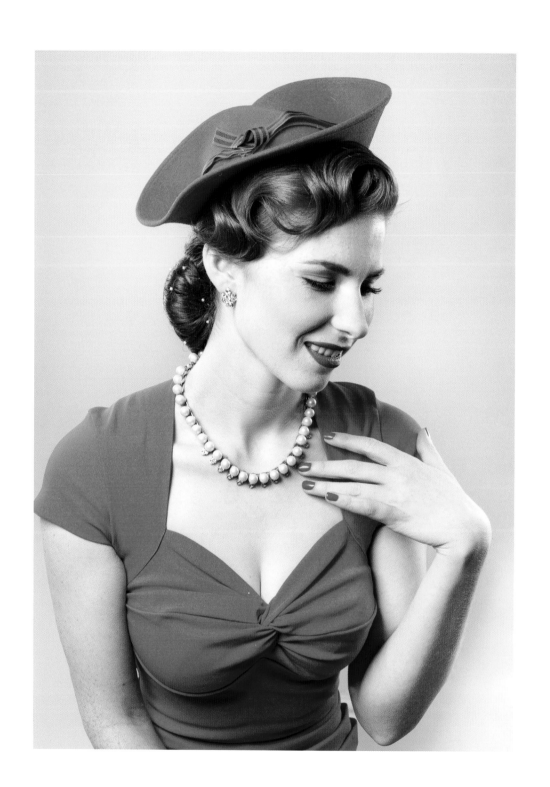

Vintage Hair Styles of the 1940s

A Practical Guide

Bethany Jane Davies

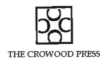

THE CROWOOD PRESS

First published in 2015 by
The Crowood Press Ltd
Ramsbury, Marlborough
Wiltshire SN8 2HR

www.crowood.com

British Library Cataloguing-in-Publication Data
A catalogue record for this book is available from the British Library.

ISBN 978 1 84797 832 5

Dedication
I would like to dedicate this book to my grandparents and to my wonderful Mum, a bookworm herself. I know she would have been so excited to see my words in print.

Cover artwork by We Are Tucano

Typeset by Sharon Dainton, The Design Co-operative Ltd.
Printed and bound in Singapore by Craft Print International

Contents

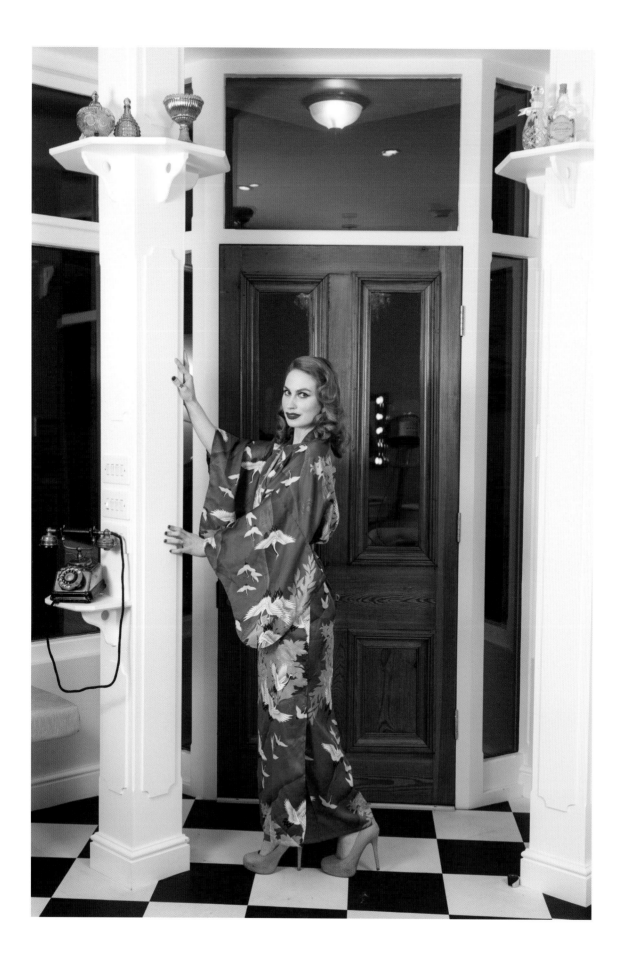

Preface: How to Use this Book

I believe that beautiful vintage hairstyles are classically flattering for any face and, hence, will always maintain their relevance within the ever-changing world of fashion trends. Classic vintage looks are accessible to everyone willing to learn the basic skills required to create them.

This book introduces and breaks down the techniques, equipment and building blocks of 1940s hairstyles using step-by-step instructions. However, as with anything creative, it is a skill that will only improve with practice, practice, practice! My advice to anyone embarking on a journey into vintage hairstyling is to pick a style to suit your skill set. Don't jump in with the most complex style involving finger waves and lots of different elements; instead, build up an arsenal of skills as you go along.

Should a style not turn out quite right, do not give up; keep experimenting until you find what works for you and your hair. Hairstyling is not a 'one size fits all' exercise; however, with a basic understanding of the concepts of preparation, correct setting methods, brushing out and styling, you will acquire the skills necessary to succeed. By using this book, you will be able to learn what works best for you and your clients. Furthermore, you will be fully equipped to adapt accordingly to any vintage style and, as a result, confidently tailor the style so that it is most flattering and enhances your beauty.

Within the methods, techniques and how-to sections, I have added a series of troubleshooting tips to help rectify common problems you may encounter while recreating the looks outlined in this book. You will not have the same hair type, length or cut as all the models in the book, but that should not stop you achieving these styles. Shorter silhouettes can be created with long hair and short hair can be formed into waves, rolls and many up styles. Notes for adapting the style to your hair can be found in the tips section below each style.

Left: The home of classic coiffeurs – the author's Vintage Beauty Parlour is popular with clients in search of an authentic vintage look. (www.bethanyjanedavies.com)

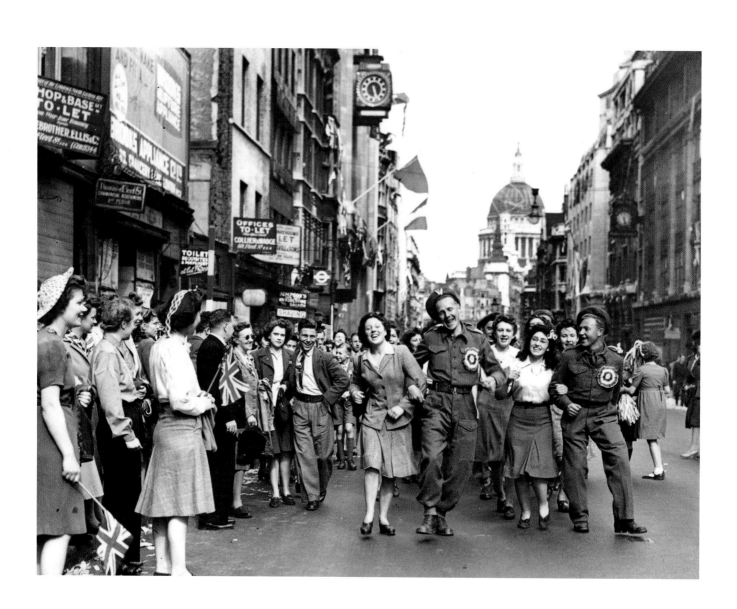

Chapter 1
Hair in the 1940s

History of the 1940s and its Effect on Hairstyles

To truly understand why certain hairstyles came into fashion during the 1940s, one must consider the social circumstances of the time; notably, the after-effects of the Second World War, the influential stars of the silver screen and the legacy of post-war recovery.

Hitler's Third Reich invaded Poland on 1 September 1939; two days later, Britain and France declared war on Germany. The nations engaged in battle were forced to channel their limited resources into the war effort. In the UK, boats that had been used previously to import goods were commandeered for military purposes; therefore, importing any goods considered non-essential became virtually impossible. Food, chemicals, metals, fabrics, soap ... they all became scarce. Keeping Britain's armed forces at war with the Germans yielded a period of austerity that impacted on Britain deeply throughout the 1940s. This factor and the lack of certain products used in hair styling would have a lasting influence on British, and indeed global, hairstyles.

In 1941 the systematic aerial bombing of Britain's key strategic cities and ports, known as the Blitz, began in earnest and brought the war directly to the doorsteps of the British people. By June 1941 fabric was in such short supply that clothing was rationed and women were obliged to 'make do and mend', fixing, tailoring and altering whatever clothing they already had. Fabric was a much-

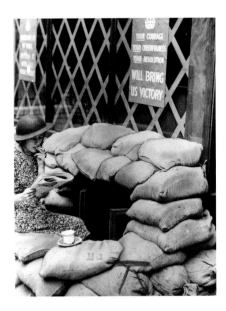

Lady taking a break during the 'Blitz'.

prized commodity not to be wasted on flimsy fashion, but style finds a way to carry on.

In December 1941, the government announced that all unmarried women between the ages of 20 and 30 were to be called up to the war effort; Britain had become the first nation in history to conscript women into the armed forces. Furthermore, all citizens up to the age of 60, men and women, were required to take part in some form of national service. This meant that, more than ever before, women became active in all aspects of working and military life. They continued to carry out their existing roles, primarily in the service industry, while also filling traditional

'men's jobs'. The women who had to undertake roles previously executed by men had to dress appropriately and manage their hair in accordance with their new-found wartime roles, but this did not stop them showing off their styles.

Women conscripts found themselves in a wide variety of jobs during this period. Numerous women worked in clerical office jobs, managing all public and domestic affairs, supporting undercover and civil operations in administrative and managerial positions. Essentially, women were fundamental to keeping their country going; therefore, there was a need for them to appear formal and smart. However, some became drivers of trucks and ambulances, while others worked as nurses in war zones.

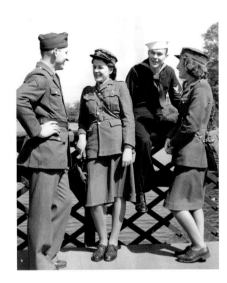

Ladies in uniform.

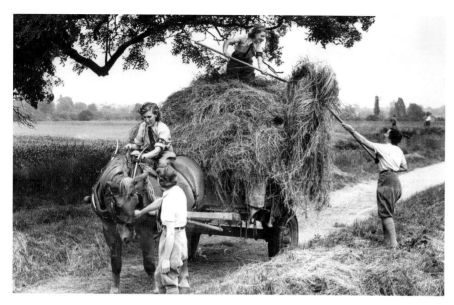

The Women's Land Army.

A large number of women undertook jobs that involved manual labour; for example, many joined the Women's Land Army (WLA), which worked the land, cultivating crops in an attempt to avoid food shortages. Others joined the Timber Corps, which involved cutting down trees and logging. These women wore robust and warm outdoor clothing and they needed to keep their hair out of their eyes so as not to impair their sight, or their ability to wield a tool.

Similarly, the women who worked in factories, munitions and steel plants worked for long periods in dangerous environments surrounded by hazardous chemicals and moving machinery. Their hair needed to be contained, as any loose or unmanaged long hair was at risk of being damaged, pulled out or causing serious harm; therefore, the wearing of hats, scarves and up-dos was frequently seen in the workplace as it was a smart way of being practical and presentable.

Turban-style scarves became an identifiable part of the working woman's wardrobe. A well-known pioneer of this style was the American cultural icon

'Rosie the Riveter', who was featured on a motivational yellow-backed poster, wearing a spotty headscarf, flexing and squeezing her bicep, alongside the slogan 'We Can Do It'. Such propaganda was intended to boost morale and keep up production. In later years, this iconic image became a symbol of feminism and female empowerment, demonstrating the extent

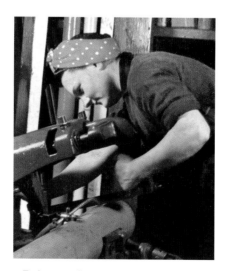

Turbans and scarves were practical for ladies in factories.

to which headscarves were engrained in the wartime culture.

Fashion adapted quickly from peacetime to wartime fashion, and became modelled more on utility clothing and active functional outfits. In the 1940s certain clothing trends achieved prominence: squared shoulders and shoulder pads were popular, as they effectively broadened the shoulders and emphasized narrow hips and narrower waists. Sharp and elegant skirts that ended just below the knee became the norm and there was an increase in the appearance of women's tailored suits, which were often minimalist with elegant straight lines. However, these styles were not readily available in high streets. Due to the rationing of fabric, new clothes were rare and the women had to double up their limited clothing as both utilitarian work wear and personal wear for all social occasions; one's work clothes might even serve as bridal wear. As the fashion silhouette became more muted, hard-wearing and, at times, somewhat plain, ladies turned to their hair as a way to add to their style; a tool they could use to express their beauty, femininity and individuality. To compensate for such plain outfits, the hairstyles became increasingly feminine and elaborate:

> 'harking back to the opulence of the Edwardian era; Joan Crawford's dressed full hair, full mouth and sculptured jackets exemplified this look.'[1]

Some women went even further by shortening their hair in the search for practicality, cutting it right down to a uniform layer, a single hair length all over the head. In 1943 this hair fashion did not go unnoticed. The publication *The Queen* was reported to have commented on the fashion, saying that:

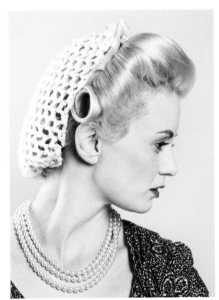

Snoods were popular due to their practicality.

Hair whilst in Uniform

Women in uniform needed hairstyles to sit neatly above the collar to stick to regulations and keep the uniform on show. In addition, the hairstyle had to work well with service caps/hats worn with certain uniforms. With so many women joining the armed forces and entering national service, the number of women in uniform grew quickly and with it grew the demand for variety. This brought about a creative spurt in styles dedicated to the uniformed woman. The hair silhouette became shorter as styles needed to be easily manageable and requiring minimal effort in an austere work environment, whilst still being attractive and feminine.

In a Universal newsreel by Ed Herlihy entitled 'News in Hairdos', style judges chose winning hairstyles for women in the armed services. The aim was to find the best coiffures for servicewomen, taking into account beauty, simplicity

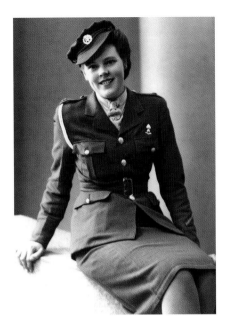

Victory rolls were popular with servicewomen.

'women have been returning more and more to short hair, abandoning the shoulder-length bob popularized by motion picture stars. Long hair, even the bob, is troublesome to keep neat, impractical for the working woman, whether she devotes her time to home defence work or is employed in the munitions or aircraft factory.'

It went on to say:

'the hair is cut to a uniform three inches all over the head, then softly waved, and the curls brushed loose. The woman who wears this type of hair can easily take care of it at home and keep it neat through a long working day.'[2]

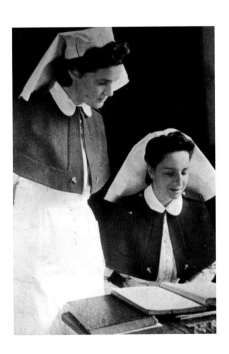

Hair needed to work well with a uniform.

and ease of grooming. Featured in this reel were some notable styles that would become influential and have inspired styles in the Step-by-Step Guide to Styles chapter of this book. One of the styles featured was the Seventh Column Hairstyle, which was a sleek style, close to the head, noted for its capacity to 'fit well under helmets (and for) work in war plants'. Next to be showcased on this reel was the Smoothie, which was deemed suitable for women engaging in civilian war work and said to be 'easy to groom, yet smart'. A final style, the Seagoing Tilt, was deemed appropriate for the Women's Royal Navy Service (popularly known as Wrens) as it was created to sit neatly under a Navy cap.

Certain techniques covered in this book, such as Victory Rolls (hair rolls at the top and front of the head), worked well with a number of hairstyles, lengths and uniforms, as the hair is swept up and away from the face to maintain a neat appearance. The Gibson Roll, hair rolls generally towards the back and bottom of the head, were particularly popular with Wrens and nurses, as their caps could sit securely on top with the roll neatly tucked away at the nape of the neck.

Many servicewomen at this time were in a hurry to marry their beau before they went to war; this meant short-notice brides. In the 1942 edition of *Modern Beauty Shop* magazine, we are told:

> 'The service bride moves fast and packs light, and her beauty program must be geared accordingly ... the service bride must not be burdened with a fancy, unmanageable hairdo.'[3]

The service bride is advised to have an easy to care for hairstyle, such as a short feather cut with a permanent wave. In this same magazine, the latest fashionable short cut is described as:

> 'the quickest way to be the prettiest bride in service. That's the demand that tops the list on the beauty programme of this June's war brides! There is little time for a leisurely beauty build up when the wedding takes place in a whirl the moment the bridegroom gets leave. That's why service brides will choose your smartest version of the feathered bob ... because it is both practical and pretty.'[4]

Looking Good and National Morale

Throughout this period, women were actively compelled to maintain their appearance for the benefit of the war effort. Both at home and at work, an attractive appearance would keep them looking and hopefully feeling their best. The British propaganda machine hoped that this positive sentiment would spread cheer amongst the domestic population and reach the troops to spur

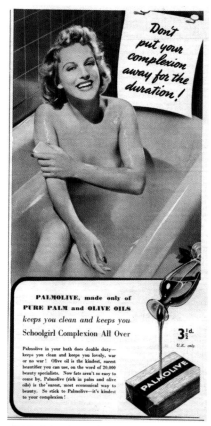

1940s Palmolive advert 'Keeps you clean and keeps you lovely war or no war'.

them on and give them something else to fight for. Throughout society, it was considered a woman's duty to keep up appearances in order to boost morale, thereby coining the phrase, 'Beauty is your duty'. Yardley, a Royal warranted beauty products and soaps company of London, truly highlighted this sentiment by running a series of wartime advertisements in the period 1942–1943 with the following tag-line: 'Put your best face forward ... To work for victory is not to say goodbye to charm. For good looks and good morale are the closest of allies.' The Yardley adverts featured a series of ladies working for the war effort: a Wren, a nurse and a factory worker, each with their own patriotic

message. Two of these messages were: 'we must see that our private troubles are not mirrored in our faces' and 'must guard against surrender to personal carelessness'.

Austerity and War: The Seed of Ingenuity

As the war continued, women found they were increasingly unable to acquire their usual hair and make-up supplies and brands. The Smith Victory Corp, a supplier of hairpins, launched a marketing campaign with the slogan 'Uncle Sam Needs the Steel'. The Vicky Victory Kit, a much sought-after wartime box of hairpins, stated on the box:

> Your hair aid warden says! Save steel, use your victory hair kit again and again! Take it to the beauty salon every time you go![5]

Out of necessity, ingenious methods were adopted by women during these times in order to keep up appearances and continue to put their best face forward. Pipe cleaners and old rags cut into strips were easier to acquire and proved to be the perfect tools for creating the popular curled styles in the absence of an iron curler or rollers. Simple water and sugar solutions were used as a setting lotion, making the hair more

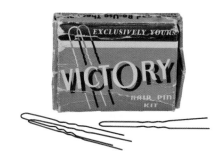

The 'Victory' hair pin kit encouraged thriftiness.

pliable and, as shampoo was in short supply, ladies began washing their hair with Lux flakes, a brand of washing powder used for laundry. Lemon was used as a rinse to brighten blonde hair and remove oil and grease, whilst vinegar was used to cleanse the scalp and give brunette locks extra shine. There are many examples of resourceful home-made 1940s recipes for hair and make-up products, many of which would still stand up against their modern, shop-bought equivalents. See the 'Home-made Lotions and Potions' section for a whole host of make-at-home beauty recipes.

Ingenuity also came in the form of military research. The Second World War heralded the birth of commercial hairspray, which emerged as a by-product of US government research into

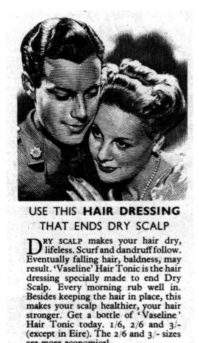

USE THIS **HAIR DRESSING** THAT ENDS DRY SCALP

DRY SCALP makes your hair dry, lifeless. Scurf and dandruff follow. Eventually falling hair, baldness, may result. 'Vaseline' Hair Tonic is the hair dressing specially made to end Dry Scalp. Every morning rub well in. Besides keeping the hair in place, this makes your scalp healthier, your hair stronger. Get a bottle of 'Vaseline' Hair Tonic today. 1/6, 2/6 and 3/- (except in Eire). The 2/6 and 3/- sizes are more economical.

PS. Don't forget to use 'Vaseline' Soapless Shampoo, 4D a packet

Vaseline HAIR TONIC

Advert for Vaseline Hair Tonic.

the development of spray cans designed to help troops to apply insect repellent evenly in an attempt to prevent malaria. The result was a pressurized aerosol can, similar to the hairspray cans we use today. However, it wasn't really until after the war that the beauty industry would pick up on the commercial opportunity to produce sticky, hard-hold, resin-based hair spray to support the curls and waves that women wanted to achieve.

Post-War Styles

Without the constraints of war, women could choose between a longer or shorter haircut out of desire rather than necessity. Soon after the end of the war in 1945, some products started to return to the market. With the relief of a return to peace, some women allowed their hair to grow longer, which brought about a trend for elegant up styles with lots of height during the immediate post-war period. These styles required more length, and classic styles became popular, such as the chignon or topknot.

The latter half of the 1940s saw a move away from utility clothing, as increasingly luxurious fabrics made their way back to prominence. The square shoulders and shorter skirts of the war era were replaced by a softer, more feminine look, exemplified by Christian Dior's New Look silhouette. This silhouette had elegant, sweeping, longer skirts with pleats and decorative folds. These skirts used large amounts of fabric, which would have been unheard of during wartime thrift. The look featured cinched-in waists and rounded shoulders, instead of the wartime trend for square ones. The New Look silhouette was incredibly popular and tended to be accompanied by shorter hairstyles. Smaller hats and caps became more prevalent with this new silhouette, which again lent themselves to a shorter, smoother hairstyle.

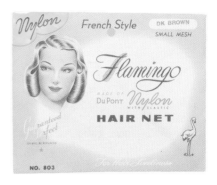

1940s hair net advert displaying the popular 'Pageboy' style.

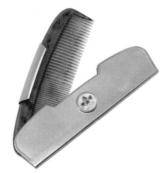

1940s hair comb.

Towards the end of the decade, hair lengths dared to go even shorter and certain styles started to incorporate looser, softer curls and waves with styles such as the Pageboy. This tendency towards soft waves, rather than tight curls, would see out the 1940s and inspire the hair fashionistas of the 1950s. The *Harpers Bazaar Folio of Fashion and Beauty* published in winter 1949 contained an article entitled 'Short Cuts to Beauty', which really highlights this shift. This article showcased a series of smooth and more relaxed styles focusing on 'simplicity' and 'sophistication', a philosophy not too dissimilar to that of wartime. However, late 1940s hairstyle trends focused on sleeker, more minimalistic versions of the early 1940s styles, with the curls more brushed out and with fewer intricacies than previously. A popular hairstyle mentioned in this article is the French

Cut: a short simple crop for someone with straight hair, possibly accompanied by 'smooth cherubic curls, brushed neatly from a diagonal parting'.

Hair Icons of the 1940s

Women in the 1940s were inspired and entranced by the high glamour, allure and sheer magic of the era's popular film stars. Television was a rarity in the home so going to the pictures was extremely popular. Ladies flocked to the cinema even during the war and, at a shilling a go, it was affordable entertainment for the masses. The glitz and glamour of the big screen was exciting and provided a welcome escape from the conflict that had the whole nation in its grip.

Why stay in when you could lose yourself watching Hedy Lamarr and Judy Garland in *Ziegfeld Girl* or Rita Hayworth and Fred Astaire in *You Will Never Get Rich*? To your cinema-goer, these icons were beautiful, inspiring, exciting and, at times, radical. The ladies wanted to be these women and the men wanted them on their arm. It was said:

> 'The development of cinema in the 1930s and 1940s set stars out on display in the same way as the latest fashions could be seen in the magically lit windows of department stores.'[6]

Hair trends amongst working women in the early 1940s were affected by some of the same practicalities familiar to modern women, such as safety in the workplace and ease of styling due to time constraints. However, that wasn't going to stop them aspiring to be like their hair icons on the silver screen!

Proof of the effect these stars had on everyday women's fashion is evident in the political and social furore caused by Veronica Lake and her 'peek-a-boo'

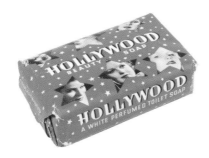

hairstyle. In cinemas across the globe, women admired her smooth, sweeping locks that obscured her right eye in a tantalizing manner. In response, the US government took it upon itself to release a public information video entitled 'Safety Styles', stating that Veronica's signature look, emulated by countless ladies, was 'entirely out of place in a war

production plant' and that wayward hair interrupted work and wasted valuable time. The video shows a new style, stating that the star 'decided to put glamour in its new wartime place and face the world with both eyes in the clear'. The hair is rolled up and away from the face in a 'simple, becoming fashion' featuring a Victory roll and small chignon bun at the back. This look was named the Victory Style.

The Top Six Hair Icons

Certain icons created a lasting impression of the true nature of 1940s glamour: distinctive, simple elegance. Depending on where you lived, certain 1940s stars were more pervasive than others. The hairstyles of those listed

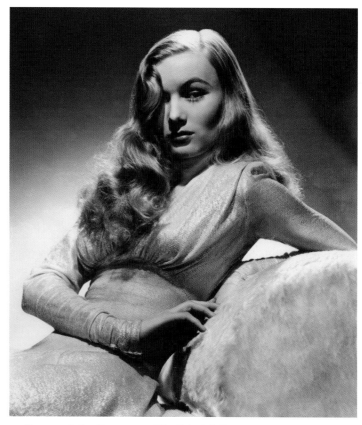

Veronica Lake. (Paramount/The Kobal Collection/Hurrell, George)

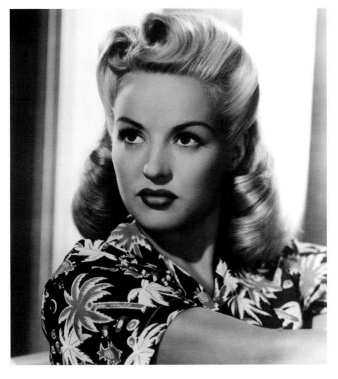

Betty Grable. (20th Century Fox/The Kobal Collection/Powolny, Frank)

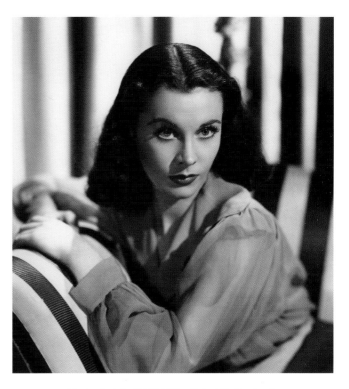

Vivien Leigh. (MGM/The Kobal Collection)

below are consistently requested by my UK clients and are extremely popular. For these top six iconic looks, it is their image and memorable style that continue to inspire modern-day vintage enthusiasts worldwide and, indeed, any student of fashion.

VERONICA LAKE

Veronica Lake's style consists of a wide, heavy side part with a distinctive S-wave sweeping down her forehead and seductively covering her right eye. There is no volume at the roots of the hair and the curls in the lengths of the hair begin below the jawline, leaving a smooth crown. Her curls are very soft and have a brushed-out effect. In some pictures the waves are fluffy and textured; in others the hair is almost completely straight with just a hint of a wave. Veronica Lake was also photographed with Victory

Rolls and the US government-sanctioned Victory Style.

Veronica Lake received her big break in the 1941 war drama *I Wanted Wings*. Although she has many film credits to her name, she is mostly remembered more for her iconic tumbling locks than her acting prowess. Peering out from behind her long blonde hair, she created an aura of mystery and allure, which made her the queen of the film noir genre in the 1940s. She was perfectly cast as the sultry vamp.

The November 1941 edition of *Life* magazine described *I Wanted Wings* as follows:

'the moment when an unknown actress named Veronica Lake walked into camera range and waggled a head of long blond hair at a suddenly enchanted public ... Veronica Lake's hair has been acclaimed by men, copied by girls, cursed by their mothers, and viewed with alarm by moralists.'[7]

The article goes on to describe the style that would become known as the 'strip-tease' and 'bad-girl' style.

Today, this style is frequently requested by vintage brides and ladies wanting a classic vintage style full of allure. Perhaps there is a little 'bad-girl' in all of us ...

BETTY GRABLE

Betty Grable was a musical film star and pin-up girl who began her career as a chorus line dancer during the 1930s. Betty's first leading role in a major Hollywood film was in *A Yank in the RAF* with Tyrone Power in 1941.

Betty's beauty and wholesome charm made her popular with both cinema audiences and troops, with her biggest

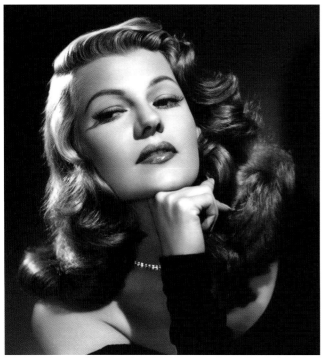

Rita Hayworth. (Columbia/The Kobal Collection/Coburn, Bob)

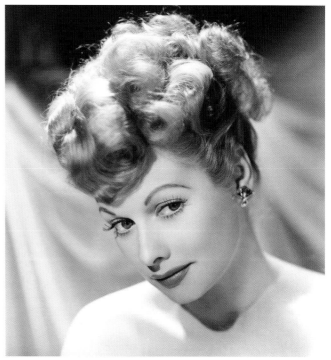

Lucille Ball. (MGM/The Kobal Collection)

hits occurring during the war.

Betty wore her hair in a number of ways, but her signature look was an upswept style with lots of height and a mass of blonde curls, which were sometimes sculpted and other times fluffy. She wore her hair down for certain shoots, but she also favoured a half-up style, tending to roll the front up into rolls or pin curls with the back of the hair down in various styles. One of the most requested styles is this image of Betty, which features smooth Victory Rolls and a pageboy-style curl at the back of the head.

VIVIEN LEIGH
Described as the perfect English rose, British-born Vivien Leigh won two Academy Awards and also cinema audiences' hearts for her performance as Scarlett O'Hara in *Gone with the Wind* in 1939. In 1940 she went on to star in

the tangled and tragic love story *Waterloo Bridge* with Robert Taylor, in which she plays ballerina Myra. The film, which opens after Britain's declaration of the Second World War, was another success.

Vivien frequently wore her brunette locks in a signature centre parting (or close to centre) with her hair brushed into soft, smooth waves. Those waves swept from Leigh's crown and down the front of her head, while the back was kept very sleek and close to the head with soft waves at the ends. Her style was simple, understated and classic, accentuating her natural beauty and framing her stunning looks.

RITA HAYWORTH
Rita Hayworth, who was born Margarita Carmen Casino, underwent a huge hair makeover before hitting the big time. Her dark locks were lightened to the

fiery red for which she was so famed; she also endured a painful course of electrolysis to make her hairline higher. Rita's lush hair, generally worn down and parted to one side with locks flowing down, her flawless skin and electric aura of sexuality made her a star.

Hayworth's biggest hit was a film noir classic released in 1946, in which she plays the eponymous femme fatale Gilda. The film by the same name features one of the most notorious introduction scenes, in which the character of Munson introduces his surprised friend Johnny to his new wife. Upon entering the room, Munson asks Gilda, 'Are you decent?' The camera cuts to a close-up of Hayworth, seductively flipping her mane of red hair back and with twinkling eyes and a wide smile she exclaims 'Me?!' After a long pause, Gilda states, 'Sure, I'm decent'.

The following year, Rita featured in

The Lady from Shanghai. For this role, her trademark red flowing locks were cut short and dyed platinum blonde. The film was a huge flop at the box office, and its failure was attributed largely to the massive change in Rita's trademark image.

Rita's tumbling locks continue to be one of the vintage styles most requested by my clients, with the publicity shot from *Gilda* being the most popular inspiration image for 1940s hair.

LUCILLE BALL

'At least once in his life, every man is entitled to fall madly in love with a gorgeous redhead.'

Lucille Ball

In 1941 Lucille Ball starred in the musical comedy film *DuBarry Was a Lady* with Gene Kelly, for which her hair was dyed the rich, flaming red that was to become her trademark. Lucille's styles featured a lot of height and typically consisted of sculpted or fluffy curls atop her head with less volume at the sides. Her luscious hair fell in smooth rolls, sometimes swept up into Victory Rolls with a fluffy textured fringe, although it is the glamorous, dramatic up-styles for which she was best known.

Lucille Ball signed with MGM in 1942 and would go on to become one of classic Hollywood's greatest beauties; she went on to enjoy one of Hollywood's longest careers on the silver screen and, eventually, television with her hit sitcom *I Love Lucy*.

In the 1946 film *Lover Come Back*, Lucille showcased the cute horseshoe-shaped fringe that has become synonymous with her style and which she favoured well into the 1950s.

LANA TURNER

Lana Turner was discovered in a Hollywood café at the tender age of sixteen. After being signed by MGM, Lana went on to become one of Hollywood's most celebrated sex symbols.

She was the classic blonde bombshell, although she was born with auburn locks that were bleached in 1939 for a film called *Idiot's Delight*, in which she never actually starred. This new look would cement her role as a popular pin-up girl of the 1940s. Leading roles in films such as *Ziegfeld Girl* and the film noir classic *The Postman Always Rings Twice* made this stunning beauty fiercely popular with cinema audiences.

Known as the Sweater Girl for some of her more form-fitting outfits, Lana was a hair chameleon with many stunning looks. Her most common styles were a short smooth bob, a down-style with long tight curls and also defined upwardly brushed waves. Lana's stunning hair was notable as she would have very deep waves and immaculately sculpted curls.

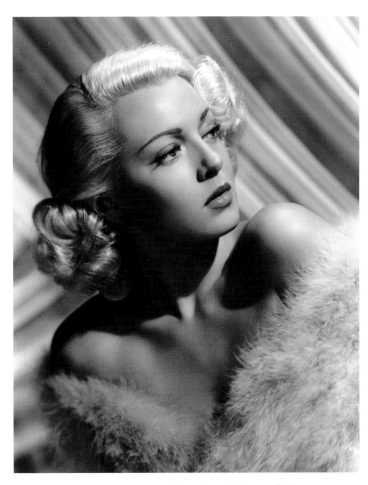

Lana Turner. (MGM/The Kobal Collection/Bull, Clarence Sinclair)

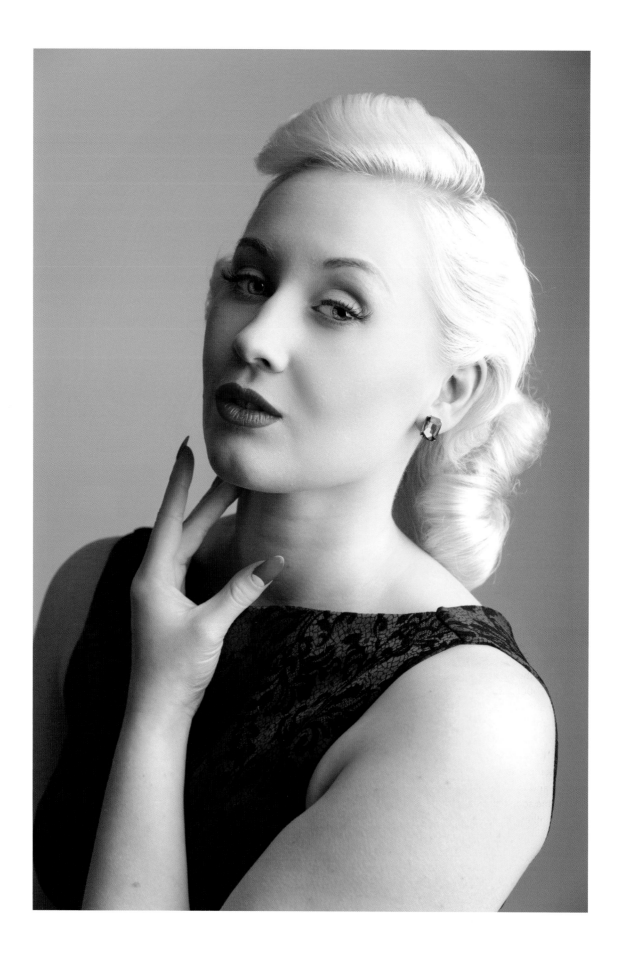

Chapter 2
Elements of 1940s Style

Women in the 1940s did not wear their hair straight or unstyled any more than they would go out without wearing underwear. Moreover, the influence of glamorous film stars, such as Lana Turner and Rita Hayworth, meant that women were increasingly choosing to colour, as well as curl their hair.

If women didn't set their hair in curls, they would have it in a braid or some variation of an up-do. Indeed, if the hair was worn up, it was most often pre-curled before being styled. The advantage of this is that once hair has been curled, it has more volume and texture, and is easier to work; therefore, curling was a clever and versatile way of keeping hair manageable for days at a time.

Hair Colouring

Men and women have been changing the colour of their hair for centuries. In ancient Egypt, records have documented the use of natural dyes, such as chamomile and indigo, while there is evidence of the plant dye henna being used since 1500BC. In the 1900s men were reported to use boot polish and ash to keep their fashionable moustaches from displaying tinges of grey.

Henna had been popular since the First World War, and even though it was acceptable in some social circles, it was frowned upon in others; consequently,

people tended to keep it a secret that they were dyeing their hair. Colouring the hair continued to grow in popularity throughout the 1920s as the flapper age burst forth and young women changed their hair colour and length. Hair was cut into fashionable bobs, inspired by starlets such as Louise Brooks and Clara Bow.

By the 1930s the fashion for dyeing one's hair declined and became stigmatized as the choice of a girl with loose morals. However, it was once again acceptable by the end of the decade. The popularity of blonde hair grew immensely due to the starlets Jean Harlow, Mae West and Ginger Rogers. Lucille Ball was not a natural redhead; she was a blonde but dyed her

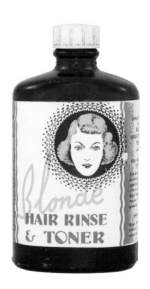

Vintage blonde hair rinse.

trademark locks using henna.

With the introduction of rationing in 1941, dye became difficult to acquire and ladies were advised to use vegetable dyes, such as indigo and henna, as an alternative to touch up their roots. They also used rinses to lighten their hair, such as chamomile and lemon.

Perming

A permanent wave is a chemical process used to create lasting curls or waves in the hair. Perming is the application of a chemical solution that changes the structure of the hair shaft, setting the hair into the desired shape with curlers or rods. Permanent waves were used as the effects were long-lasting, meaning that women could recreate their desired styles with fewer trips to the salon and obtain fashionable styles with less effort.

The first perming machine was invented by Karl Nessler. The hair was set around metal rods connected to a machine with an electric heating device. Caustic soda was then applied and the hair was left to heat for a long period of time. It is said the first two attempts burned off all of his long-suffering wife's hair, but by 1909 the method had been improved somewhat and was used as a hair curling method. In 1938 Arnold F. Willatt invented the cold wave – the precursor to the modern perm. Using neither machines nor heat, this method was a breath of fresh air for women who wanted to add a permanent curl to their hair and give their sets staying power.

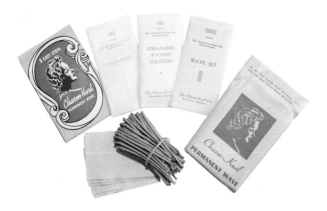

1940s home perm kit.

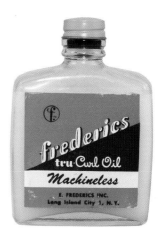

Machineless perming solution.

Perming was very popular in the 1940s and perms were used in conjunction with wet sets to create lasting curl. Hairspray was not widely available and nor were heated hair appliances, so the ladies of the time jumped at any chance to achieve longevity with their hairstyles. Even during the war, women still got their hair permed, although not always with the best results, as described by this school teacher:

'My perm took from 9.30 to 12.30, but I don't think I quite like the way she has done it. She gave me a sort of halo of little curls, and they don't look quite right with my moon-like countenance.'

She goes on to describe another perm, which:

'has descended from the corrugated-iron stiffness into a brief and frizzy mass. Like wool.'[8]

The American company Toni was one of the first companies to release a home perm kit. The kits contained a chemical agent that was applied to the hair, which was then rolled in curlers and a neutralizing agent applied to hold the resulting curls. Pin-Up Perms home perming kit was established in 1945 with the tag line: 'This is why young stars have Pin-up Perms'. After the war, such products became more readily available to the masses so perms rose even more in popularity, as they produced a much more lasting set than rollers, rags or pin curls. It was easy to get a permed set and simple to snap it into shape.

Today, perming has decreased in popularity due to the damage it can cause to the hair. The strong chemicals can make the hair brittle and fragile. If you are considering getting a perm, experiment first with a wet pin curl set or rags to see if a stronger curling technique can give your hair more hold. Always get your perm done professionally and speak to a hairdresser to see if a perm is the right option for your hair type.

Curls and Waves

This section covers the primary components of 1940s style, the combination of which form the basis of the archetypal 1940s hairstyle. These are Rolls, Curls, Waves, Pompadours, Braids, Hairpieces and Fringes. Once you know these components, you can recreate pretty much any 1940s style.

Most 1940s styles begin with some form of hot or wet curl; the curl is pinned to the head in order to set, in other words completely cool or dry. Once set, the curls are released, whereupon they can be brushed out to form a desired shape, be that a smooth wave, or a fluffy or sculptured curl.

Curls move around each other falling into a spiral corkscrew shape, which, in turn, creates hair volume. Mastering the skill of hair curling is undoubtedly the most powerful tool for anyone wishing to create these vintage styles. The curls set in the hair form the core framework for building any 1940s period hairstyle.

As well as being used as a method for curling the hair when wet, pin curls are used as a decorative feature when rolled

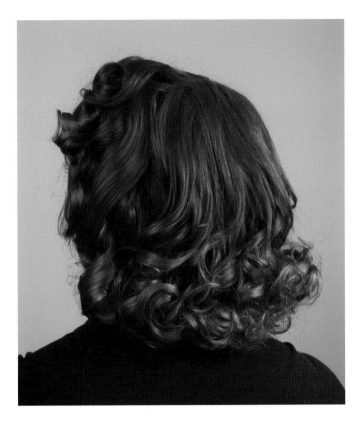

Hair styled into curls.

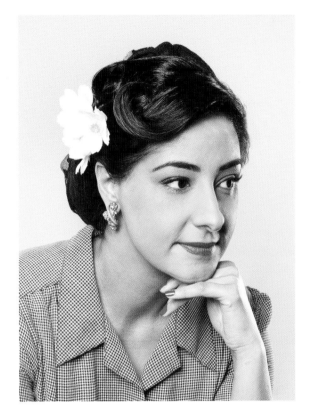

Dry pin curls.

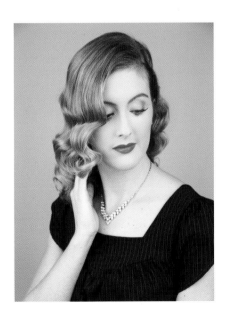

Hair styled into waves.

in dry hair. The section of hair is rolled around fingers to form a circle or free form at the end of the hair and is then pinned to the head.

A wave is a smooth finish that creates a continuous S shape in the hair and was a prominent staple during the 1940s. The style is created when sections of hair, curled in opposite directions, are brushed together. The two oppositely rolled strands meet, create ridges and flow from one side to another along the hair's length, thus creating an unbroken wave. The wave gives depth and definition to what would otherwise be a flat section of hair; therefore, the wave becomes a focal point of the hairstyle as the light catches the wave differently throughout the S shape.

Rolls

Rolls were a consistent feature of 1940s hairstyles. Outlined below are some of the most prevalent rolls used during this period and step-by-step instructions can be found in Chapters 6 and 7.

- A Victory Roll is an instantly recognizable 1940s style or component thereof, where the hair is rolled up into tunnel-shaped curls, swept away from the face, generally pinned towards the top and sides of the head. Victory rolls were a common feature of many 1940s hairstyles and were popular as they can be styled into many different lengths. A hairstyle could feature just one large Victory roll or several smaller rolls, meaning that many variations of styles can incorporate this type of roll. The versatile Victory Roll could be assimilated on the side, top or the back of the head and feature in smooth up-dos and fluffy pin curl sets. Interestingly, the

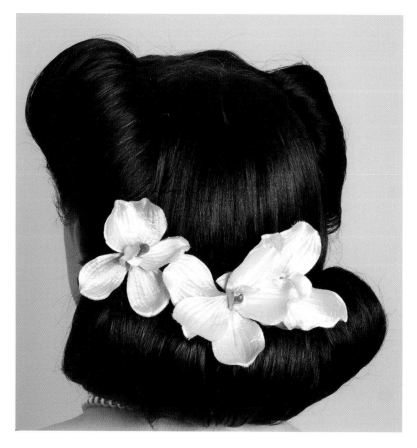

Gibson Roll.

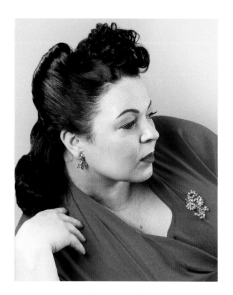

Victory Roll.

Victory Roll is said to have gained its name from the fighter plane manoeuvres of the Second World War, as its swirls and rolls mimicked the contrails left when pilots looped and rolled the planes following a successful mission. Thus, the name Victory Roll was coined by patriotic ladies and its name will have no doubt have added to its appeal throughout the 1940s.

- The Gibson Roll is one style, or component thereof, in which the hair is rolled upwards at the nape of the neck, usually making the neck visible. Ladies were known to tie an old stocking around their head, rolling the hair over it, to create one continuous roll or band of hair almost all the way around the head, covering the stocking at the front with more rolls or curls.

- The Pageboy, a smooth roll, rolled downwards and under, is almost the opposite of the Gibson Roll, going all the way around the back of the head. This style results in a sleek back

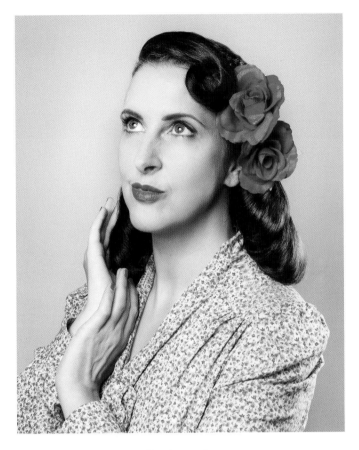

Pageboy style.

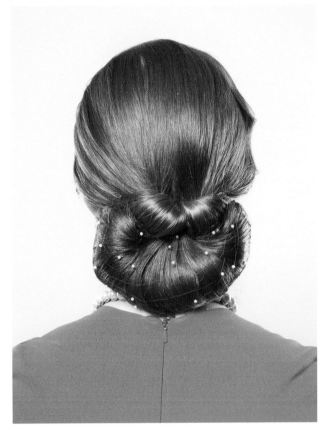

Chignon.

of the head and profile, with a soft bump around the nape, and was very popular throughout the 1940s and well into the 1950s.

To help create rolls, pre-curling the hair will help provide extra volume and also bend the hair in the desired direction, making it easier to work with and mould into shape.

Buns and Chignons

The chignon is a roll or knot of hair worn at the back of the neck. This chic style typically has upswept sides and sits in a low bun, but it has many variations. It

was an easy and practical style when women wanted their hair kept neat and out of the way when at work, but it could also be dressed up for evening elegance.

Pompadours

The Pompadour is a style in which the hair is swept upwards from the face and worn high away from the forehead, not unlike a quiff. It can be smooth, waved or curly and is generally swept up at the sides. Like rolls, volume is important in creating the Pompadour style and this can be achieved by back-brushing, stuffing and also pre-curling the hair.

Braids, Hairpieces and Extensions

Braids were a very popular way of styling the hair during the 1940s. Most commonly, these were formed from the individual's own hair; however, there are many examples of styles incorporating a switch, a braided hairpiece of either synthetic or human hair, which would be pinned into the individual's hair in order to appear natural. Contrasting colours of hair were also used in some extravagant pieces and others had adornments within the switch, braided with pearls, scarves or ribbons for added effect.

Hairpieces and extensions were

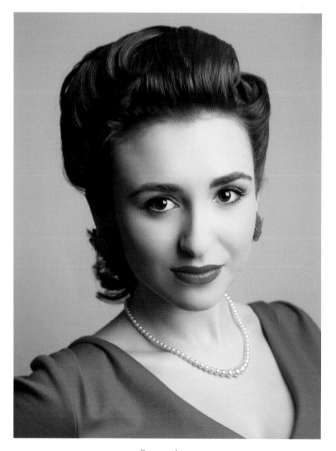

Pompadour.

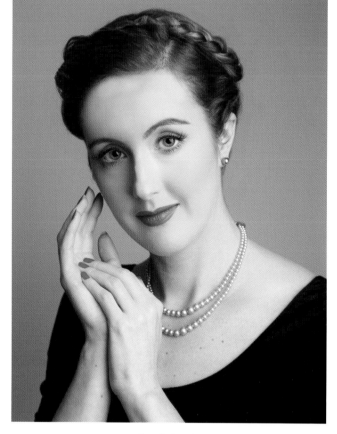

Braided style.

generally very popular throughout the decade. An article in *Colliers* magazine in July 1941 exclaimed that 'bangs on a comb, stately coronets (a crown) of braided hair, luscious chignons mounted on hairpins, and gleaming cascade bobs on an elastic have gone to the heads of the nation'. Furthermore, an advert for June Hair Products states: 'However long or short your hair may be, added hair means added styles and added charm.' They were right. Modern fashions still focus on adding volume and bounce to give the effect of healthy, youthful hair.

So, which type of hair is best? Real hair is best for any pieces that require curling, as heat will melt synthetic hair. It is also very hard to wet set or dye synthetic hair. In contrast, synthetic hair is perfect for braids as it stays smooth, keeps its shape and it is very useful for stuffing as it is hygienic and inexpensive.

Fringes

In the 1940s silhouette, fringes – known as bangs in North America – would often be pulled away from the face.

However, certain looks did incorporate a number of fringe styles and the 1940s fringe tended to be carefully sculpted. If the fringe fell down over any part of the face or forehead, it was shaped in order to have a defined edge and contained waves, rolls, fluff curls or lots of small curls.

Fringes can be created in long hair by rolling the hair around a sausage-shaped 'Rat' and pinning at the sides. Curling long hair into small ringlets and pinning at the top of the forehead can also give the illusion of a fringe.

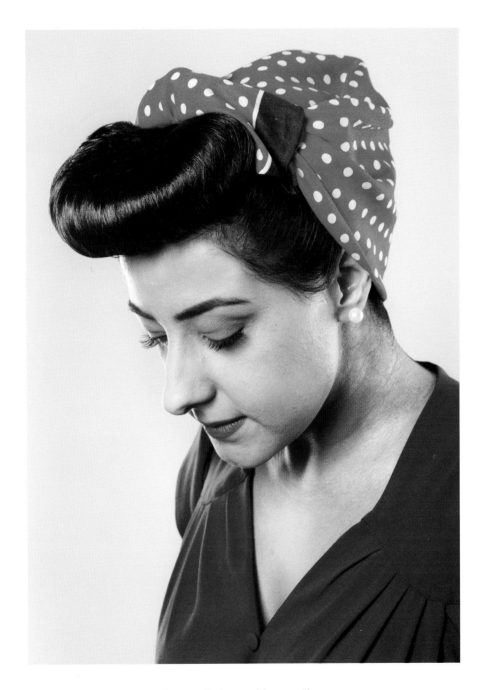

Fringe rolled around foam stuffing.

1940s Hair Accessories

Ladies in the 1940s wore a large variety of hair accessories for practical and decorative purposes. In summer 1947 a lifestyle magazine reported on their popularity:

'A wide taffeta ribbon that ties in a bustle bow adds femininity. Braids belong to any age but must be manipulated to make the most of your face. Flowers, real or make-believe, turn into evening chignons. Scarf rings, pearls, and pins lead new lives on top of beautifully groomed heads.'[9]

A whole host of options are available for matching with your outfit or personalizing your style, and making it suitable for day or evening wear. Use accessories to refresh your set on day two or three when your curls may have dropped a little or to cover any flaws in a style that hasn't turned out as well as planned.

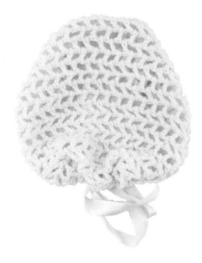

Snood.

Snoods

A snood is a bag/net that covers and holds the hair at the back of the head. Snoods tend to be knitted, crocheted or made of net and lace; however, they can also be fashioned from scarves and fabric.

The most common way to wear a snood is to pin it at the crown of the head with the hair at the back tucked neatly inside. The front of the hair can be styled in a variety of ways.

This is an easy and practical style that, traditionally, kept the hair in place whilst working in a factory. As an accessory, a snood works wonders for protecting the hair from the elements or creating a quick, authentic style on a bad hair day. For evening wear, try a pearled snood or decorate by adding flowers.

If you find your hair peeks through the snood, try wearing a hairnet underneath in a similar shade to your hair. Make sure the snood is the right length for your hair, and take care to pin it higher if you have shorter hair, as a baggy snood is not attractive. If you have very fine hair, pull some extra hair forward to form Victory Rolls – this will give you

nice thick rolls at the front. If needed, you can clip in a few extension wefts at the back and use these to bulk out the snood.

Turbans

Use a turban to cover your pin curl set as you go about your day for a slice of 1940s glamour. Purchase a turban in

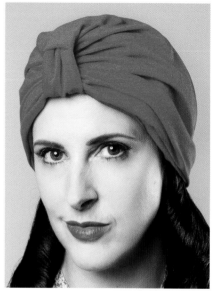

Turban.

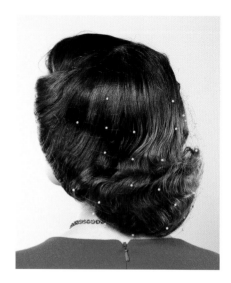

Hairnet.

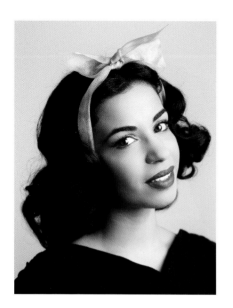

Ribbon.

your favourite colour or follow the turban tutorial and make your own out of a scarf or strip of fabric.

Your turban can be worn with a fringe or all of you hair tucked away. Accessorize with flowers tucked in at the front or brooches for added sparkle.

Hairnets

In addition to the practical uses of protecting your pin curl set or supporting the hair, nets can also be used for decorating your style. Nets can be found adorned with pearls and diamanté and look beautiful stretched over a chignon or pageboy haircut.

Combs and Clips

Used to securely hold your style in place, combs and hair clips are a perfect way of

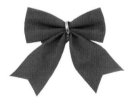

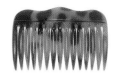

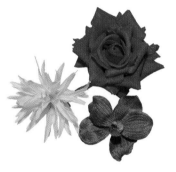

Hair accessories.

adding decoration to your style. Glue flowers, pearls or jewels to your comb to create a unique hair ornament.

Flowers

Flowers finish off a style and are a beautiful addition to any vintage style. A whole host of flowers can be found at your local garden centre or craft shop, and you can create your own with a hot glue gun and some hairpins or curl clips.

When adding to your style, ensure that the flowers blend well rather than just sticking out from the hair. Remember, they are also useful for covering flaws in a style.

Ribbons and Bows

Ribbons and bows are great accessories. Weave ribbons through plaits or tie

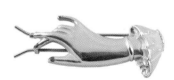

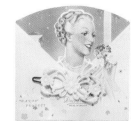

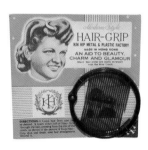

around the head to brighten up a daytime style. Bows can be attached to kirby grips, allowing them to blend easily with many styles.

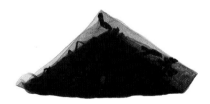

Scarves

Add some colour to your daytime style with a scarf tied in a bow or dressed into plaits. Use your scarf to create a snood or turban and style the front of your hair into rolls or pin curls for a quick hair fix.

Hats

Hats were an extremely popular accessory in the 1940s. The silhouette of the era, which often featured a smooth crown and a halo of curls, was dictated by the popularity of the hat as this shape meant the hat would sit correctly on the head.

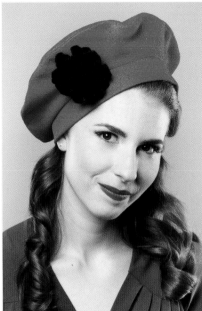

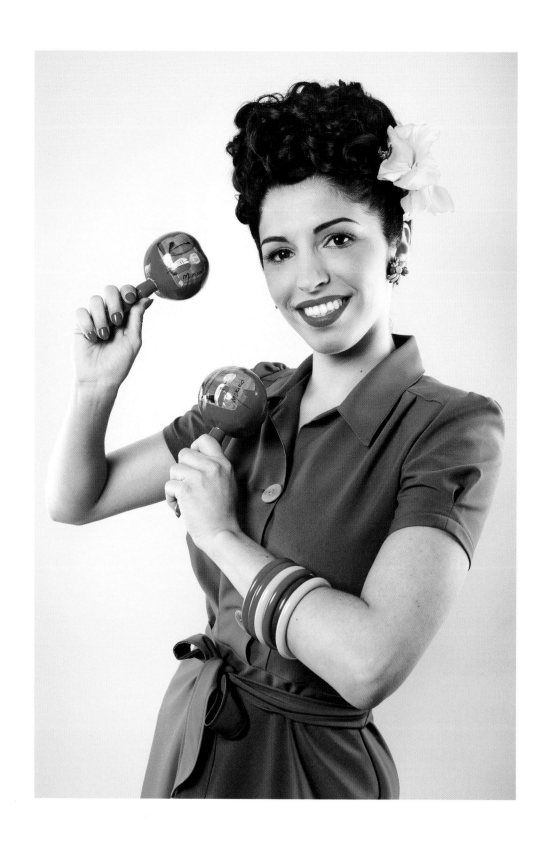

Chapter 3
Before You Style

Products

Hairspray

Hairspray holds your finished style in place, supports your curls and is available in many different strengths.

Misting your hair with a flexible-hold hairspray as you style will help to shape and sculpt your hair, and also makes it more pliable when brushing out wet sets.

Make sure you don't hold the can too close to the hair as this distributes the spray unevenly and makes the hair wet. To smooth and finish styles, spray the hair with a fine mist and smooth down any stray hairs with your fingers or very gently with a bristle brush or comb.

Heat Protector

This thermal spray is used prior to styling to protect your tresses from heat damage, especially when using high-heat stylers such as tongs or straighteners. It also helps hold and set the curl for longer with all types of curling methods. Protection is particularly important when styling chemically treated hair, as it will be weaker and more susceptible to damage.

Pomade

Pomade is essential for vintage styles. It is fabulous for helping sculpt the hair, smooth flyaway hairs and adding shine, resulting in a polished finish. Pomade also has the benefit of holding the shape of curls once the set is brushed out.

Take a small amount of pomade and work it through your hands, smoothing and shaping with your fingers to distribute it through your hair. Keep replenishing the pomade on your fingers as you work through the style. There are numerous different brands to try; some have lighter formulations than others, depending on your hair type and thickness.

Setting Lotion

If you are doing a wet set, a setting lotion should be used. Setting lotions in the 1940s were often home-made and recipes used stale beer, quince seeds, flax seeds and sugar syrup, to name but a few ingredients.

Today there is a variety of brands and types available and they can be used either mixed with water or on their own. Setting lotion makes the hair more malleable and easier to manipulate, holding the hair in place as it sets. It also helps give the finished style more longevity once the hair has been brushed out into the desired finish. See Chapter 9 for instructions for making your own setting lotion.

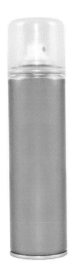

Hairspray.

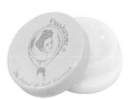

Vintage pomade.

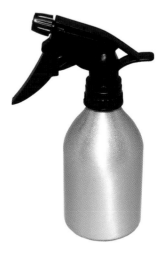

Spray bottle.

Dry Shampoo

Dry shampoo is available in spray or powder form and is great for prolonging the life of sets by absorbing oil from the roots. It also adds texture to the hair, thereby enabling it to be rolled and sculpted with ease if you have silky hair or it is freshly washed.

Back-combing Spray/Powder

These are perfect for adding volume to the roots of fine hair and adding texture when rolling and styling. If you want to create rolls without back-brushing, this is a must.

Tools

Brushes

Brushing and dressing out the hair is crucial when creating 1940s styles; therefore, you need a good-quality brush that is fit for purpose.

BRISTLE BRUSHES

For general styling, I recommend a brush with a mix of synthetic and boar bristles as this is perfect for back-brushing, smoothing and gently brushing out hot sets. The larger synthetic bristles detangle while the natural bristles smooth.

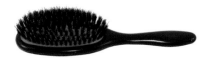

Bristle brush.

STYLING BRUSH

A stronger bristle is required when brushing out wet sets. A synthetic nylon bristle is preferable as natural bristle can cause excess frizz when brushing out pin curls, rags and other sets. A larger, vented brush with fewer teeth or a rubber pad can also help reduce frizz.

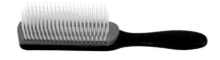

Styling brush.

DRESSING OUT BRUSH

This works well for back-brushing and smoothing the hair into rolls. Its thin width makes it useful for precision styling without disturbing other areas of the style.

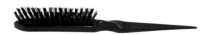

Dressing out brush.

DETANGLING BRUSH

Specially designed with flexible bristles, these brushes are ideal for removing tangles without damage prior to setting. They are also useful for tackling tangles when removing Victory Rolls or back-brushing.

   Brush out tangles when the hair is dry, before washing or wetting down with setting lotion. Never remove the tangles from your hair while it is still wet as your hair is at its weakest in this state and breakage can occur.

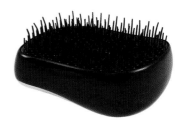

Detangling brush.

Combs

TAIL COMB

This comb is perfect for sectioning off hair and tweaking styles. Use the pointed end to section the hair for pin curls, hot sticks or rolls. The fine teeth are used to create tension on the hair before curling (also known as ribboning) and the tail end is used to tuck the ends of the hair around rollers to avoid hooked ends.

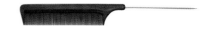

Tail comb.

DRESSING COMB

The two different widths of teeth enable you to change the tension on the hair; the thinner side has the most tension. When finger-waving, using the wider comb can be helpful for very thick hair, whilst the opposite is true for finer hair.

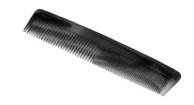

Dressing comb.

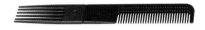

Styling and lifting comb.

STYLING AND LIFTING COMB

These combs add volume to a style by using the pronged ends to lift hair from the roots when finishing a style. They are perfect for fine hair.

Sectioning Clips

These are useful for holding the hair in place when dividing it into sections. Duckbill clips are used to help mould waves in the hair by clamping in position those you have created as you continue to work through other sections of hair.

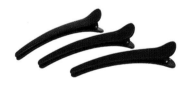

Sectioning clips.

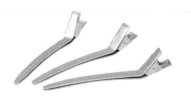

Duckbilled clips.

Pin Curl Clips

These are used for holding curls while they cool after using tongs. They are also used to hold wet pin curls in place whilst they dry. They are available in single and double prongs. The single prongs are perfect for pinning stand-up pin curls and flat pin curls in fine hair, while the double-prong clips are better for large pin curls and thicker hair.

Pin curl clips can also be used in conjunction with hairspray to shape the final style by using the clips to manipulate the shape, spraying with firm-hold spray and then removing the clips.

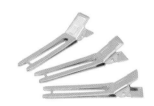

Double prong clips.

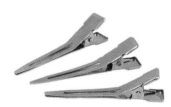

Single prong clips.

Kirby Grips

Also known as bobby pins, kirby grips are used to secure styles in place. Find grips to match your hair colour as they will be easily hidden within your hairstyle. If your hair is very slippery or thick, you can purchase coated pins that have a rougher texture, giving more hold.

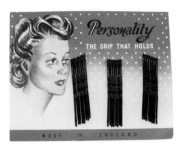

Kirby grips.

Hairpins

Hairpins are used to shape the hair and to hold wet pin curls in place. To use hairpins properly, a lever action is required. Hairpins provide a much looser hold than grips. They come in different sizes, with the larger hairpins perfect for securing chignons and the finer pins ideal for securing and shaping Victory Rolls.

For extra security in the hair, bend the ends of the pin before inserting into the hair.

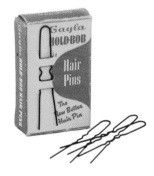

Hair pins.

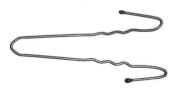

Hair pin bent for added security.

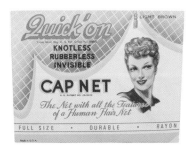
Vintage hair net.

Hairnets

These thick nets are essential for protecting your set as you sleep. Scarves can also be used, but nets allow more air to circulate around your set, which is especially important if you have thick hair or hair that takes a long time to dry. Thin 'invisinets' can be used to support your style.

Hair Combs

These are used to hold styles in place and pull back and secure sections of hair. They are perfect for controlling thick hair but also work well in finer hair, as pushing the comb towards the hairline once in the hair can create extra volume. Small, fine combs work well on thinner hair, whilst the larger combs are perfect for lots of thick hair.

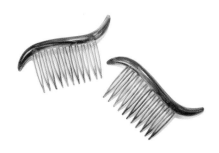
Hair combs.

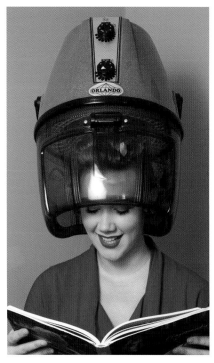
Hood dryer.

Hood Dryer or Bonnet Dryer

Hood dryers circulate warm air around your set and speed up drying time. They are available as large standing dryers with adjustable heights, bonnet dryers that are attached to a hair dryer and inflated, or small table-top models.

These are a very useful tool to have, especially in cool weather when sets take longer to dry, or when you need your set ready in a jiffy.

Stuffing and Rats

Stuffing a roll with some form of lightweight filler can help provide more body and stability. In a modern salon, one might use a sponge of the same colour as the hair; however, in the 1940s the stuffing was usually improvised out of one's own loose hair and known affectionately as a Rat, presumably after a half-asleep husband's horror at seeing

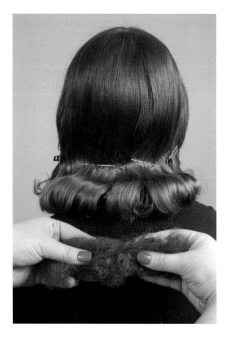
Using stuffing – step 1.

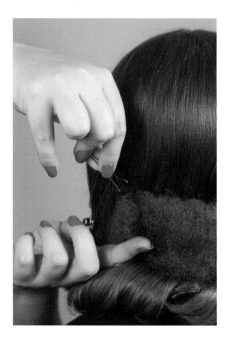
Using stuffing – step 2.

a stray, hairy one under the dressing table.

In typical make do and mend style, women would take a laddered stocking or hair net and stuff it with either more

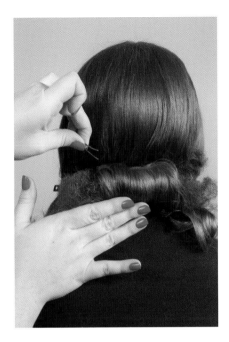

Using stuffing – step 3.

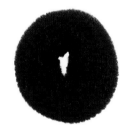

Hair doughnut.

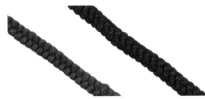

Crepe hair used for stuffing and making 'Rats'.

stockings beyond repair or with their own hair that had been dutifully collected from a hairbrush and stored in a 'hair receiver' on the dressing table. These methods can still be used today – or pop down to your local pharmacy where there are modern options, such as foam doughnuts/sausages, or crepe hair

available in a variety of colours. Old hair extensions can be also made into stuffing by rolling them in an old hairnet. Indeed, hairnets full of hair, fake or otherwise, are easier to pin than stockings.

See Chapter 8 for instructions to make your own Hair Rat.

Prepping the Hair for Styling

Keeping the Hair and Scalp Healthy

Regular brushing was considered an important element of 1940s hair care. Women were advised to get into the habit of vigorously massaging the scalp and brushing the hair for at least twenty minutes in the morning and again at night to increase the circulation and blood flow to the scalp. This was thought to encourage healthy hair growth and to distribute natural oils produced by the scalp through the hair, and:

'Not only keep the hair clean but also give the gloss and lustre that people so admire.'[10]

Today, rather than vigorous daily brushing, head massage is a perfect way to stimulate the scalp and get your blood flowing. So next time you put on a hair treatment, don't forget about your scalp.

Recipes from the 1940s for rinses, hot oil treatments and other remedies aimed at boosting hair and scalp health are available in the 'Home-made Lotions and Potions' section of this book.

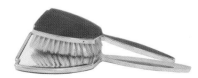

1940s Brush Set.

Virgin Hair and Chemically-treated Hair

If you use colour or any chemical treatments on your hair, you must ensure you protect and prepare your hair for styling by keeping it in good condition and by using a good-quality heat protector. Heat-protection sprays act as a barrier by absorbing some of the heat, and prevent breakages and prolong curls. Chemically treated hair can often be easier to shape and hold a curl, but it can become brittle, unhealthy and difficult to style if heavily damaged.

Hair that has never been chemically treated or dyed is called virgin hair. However, it is not always the easiest hair to style. Therefore, if you find it hard to get lasting curl in your hair – if your hair

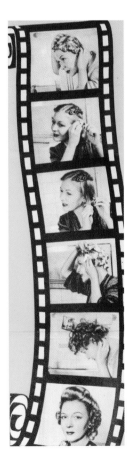

Instructions for a home perm.

is naturally very straight, for example – it is worthwhile experimenting more with wet sets as their staying power far outweighs that of hot sets.

Hair Washing

Unwashed hair is generally easier to style for most people. The more you wash your hair, the more its natural oils are stripped away. This initiates a vicious circle where the scalp works hard to replace these oils, which can make the hair appear greasy. It is advisable to reduce the number of washes to the minimum required; daily washing is ill-advised. As well as producing more oils at the roots, daily washing can lead to less lustrous locks as the ends of the hair can become overly dry. Another benefit of washing your hair less frequently is that if you dye your hair, the colour will not fade as quickly, meaning fewer top-ups at the hairdresser and ultimately more pennies in your pocket.

To help fight the urge to wash every day, try using a dry shampoo to refresh your hair and remove excess oil. In addition, on the day when you feel you must wash your hair, try an up-do instead.

As a general rule, if you are using heat, freshly washed hair is not ideal, because when your hair has been washed it is very slippery and soft from the conditioner and lack of natural oils to give it some hold. Squeaky-clean hair can slip out of pins and is notoriously hard to style. Therefore, if you are new to styling your hair into vintage looks, make your job easier and practise on one- or two-day-old unwashed hair. That bit of natural oil makes it easier to style and adds to its longevity as the curls will not drop out as quickly.

The Cut

Having the right cut for vintage styling is important. Just as in baking, having the right ingredients produces better results. A good foundation for your style is just as important as the curling and shaping. The cut you have will determine the techniques and positioning of curls in order to achieve your desired look. Keeping your hair trimmed regularly will also reduce frizzy ends when you come to brush out curl sets.

Some modern blunt haircuts, those without layers, make it more difficult to reproduce an authentic vintage look, as the 1940s woman tended to have layers in her hair. Layers are vital for imitating 1940s styles, as they allow the curls to sit naturally and give depth to the style. This is not to say that if you have a blunt cut you will not get a good result or that your cut is wrong. Hair styling is not a 'one size fits all' solution, and experimenting with different-sized rollers and curl positioning can help. With blunt cuts, the curls tend to sit in a single straight row; however, with layers and vintage cuts, the curls are staggered in several rows and at varying heights, which creates a natural U-shape around the nape.

Faking it

To create the illusion of a U shape with a blunt cut, when rolling the hair for setting put the rollers or hot sticks or other curling method in a U-shaped curve.

Use two different sizes of pin curl, roller, hot stick or rag. Form larger curls towards the bottom of the hairline around the back and sides, and smaller tighter curls towards the top of the back and sides. When brushed out, this

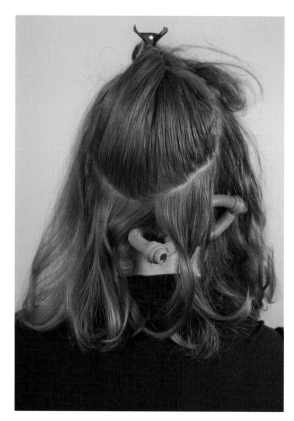

When setting the hair, section in a U-shape to fake a vintage cut.

produces curls that sit on top of each other, following the curve of the head in a U shape.

THE VINTAGE CUT

The most popular cut for women during the 1940s was the Middy Cut. Created by legendary Warner Brothers' stylist Ivan Anderson, the Middy Cut was heavily layered, with an elongated U-shaped baseline at the back and steeply slanting sides. Once hair was curled with this cut, it settled naturally into beautiful layered waves.

Compared with modern standards, 1940s hair was short. A classic Middy Cut was usually around 10cm/4ins long with less length on the sides and slightly more at the back. Adding a couple more inches in length to the back of a Middy Cut became known as the Femme Fatale. The hair baseline at the back followed the natural curve of the hairline and both the Middy and Femme Fatale allow for more curling around the back of the hair. Shorter variations of the Middy Cut, such as the Shingle and the cropped Baby Cut, focus more on curling at the top of the hair.

The Middy Cut is not really a wash-and-wear style due to the U-shaped layers that make it somewhat akin to an unstyled mullet shape. Therefore, if you seldom set it or like to put it up in a ponytail regularly, it is probably not advisable to go for the full Middy Cut; settle for a few layers instead. Before you decide to take the plunge and opt for a Middy Cut, consider how long you spend styling your hair. If you are planning to set it once or twice a week, and wish to create an authentic vintage style, this could be the cut for you.

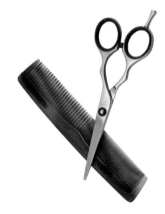

Getting the right cut.

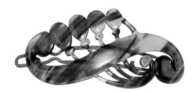

1940s hair clip.

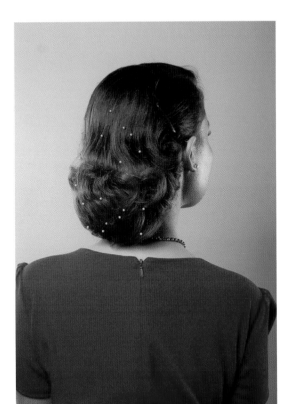

The classic 1940s silhouette was a U-shape.

HAIR LENGTH

The length of your hair will affect how long your hair holds a curl. More length adds extra weight to the hair, and with it the tendency for the curls to drop. If your hair is very long, having a few layers takes out some of the weight from the curl. In addition, wet sets tend to hold curls better.

Longer hair with a natural wave or curl can hold curl at length, but if you have fine or naturally straight hair, you may find taking a bit off the length will help give your curls more bounce and durability.

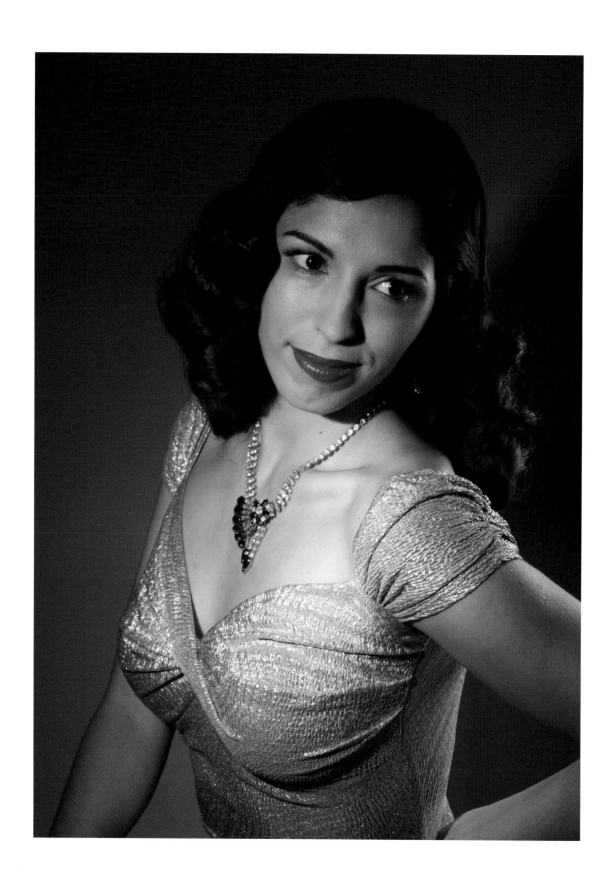

Chapter 4
Creating Curls and Rolls

Whether you plan to create your curls with heat or with water, there are key elements that are vital to all curling methods. These factors will affect the type of curl you create, how much volume is in the hair, how long your curls will hold and how easy they will be to brush out. Be sure to understand these concepts before proceeding.

In this chapter I will cover the processes needed to set your hair successfully whether you choose to set it wet or dry. For information and tips on brushing out all of the different sets please see the 'Brushing Out' chapter.

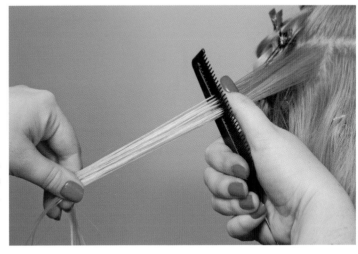

Ribboning a section before curling.

The Key Elements for Creating Curls

Tension

When curling your hair – wet or dry – tension is important. A loose roller or pin curl will lose tension and produce a weak set.

When wet setting your hair, make sure you 'ribbon' the section. This technique creates tension by forcing the hair

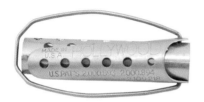

Vintage metal roller.

between the thumb and the back of the comb.

When curling with heat, ensure each section is tangle-free and held taut when rolling or tonging, with the ends neatly tucked in.

When using foam rollers, the hair should be brushed through, but you must ensure you do not squash the roller when wrapping the hair around it as this will distort the curl.

Width of Section and Curl

The width of the section is very important and has a significant effect on the outcome of your style.

For rollers (wet and dry), the general rule is to use a section of hair the same width and length as the roller being used.

For tongs, the width should also match

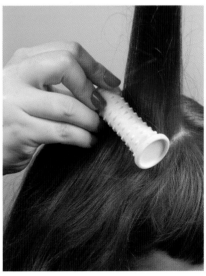

Correct sectioning for roller.

that of the tong but can be longer in length and set in tubes. The same applies to hot sticks.

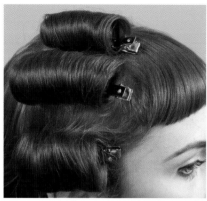

With pin curls, the bigger the section or 'base', the larger the curl will be; this is also true for rag curls.

When you are choosing what size barrel, roller or pin curl to use, think about the width of the waves you would like to create.

Here we see three widths of curl created with tongs 2cm, 3cm and 4cm wide.

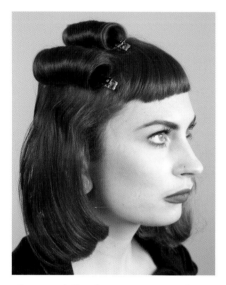

Large curl. Best for creating root volume for Victory Rolls or very smooth, brushed-out styles on hair that curls very well.

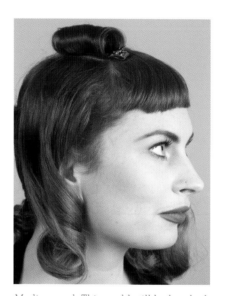

Medium curl. This could still be brushed into waves or curls that form well but may drop quickly on straight hair.

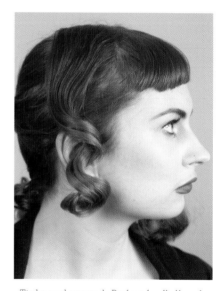

Tight curl created. Perfect for fluff curls and tight waves.

Base Direction

The base is the stationary foundation of the curl, which is the area closest to the scalp and the panel of the hair on which the roller, pin curl or hot stick sits.

Base direction is created by the angle in which the hair is pulled before the curl is set with tongs, rollers, hot sticks or pin curls. The angle at which the hair is rolled to the scalp and sits on its base determines the amount of volume a curl has and whether it is 'over directed', 'on base' or 'off base'.

On Base: Creates a strong curl with full volume. The hair is held straight up from the head and sits directly on the base of the section.

Over Directed: Creates the largest amount of volume. The hair is held and curled in the opposite direction to where the roller will sit. The rolled section of hair sits slightly forward of and above its base.

Off Base: Creates no volume at the scalp and is perfect for achieving the popular 1940s look of a smooth crown. This curl sits completely off its base, below the section. This type of curl can sit just centimetres off base or the uncurled section, or 'stem', can be longer. They are both classified as off-base curls and the stem length should be adjusted depending on the desired final result.

Ultimately, the base direction of the curl will affect the volume of the curls and the look of the final set.

Here is a hot stick set with one side set off base and the other half on base. Note the difference in the outcome.

If you are pre-curling the hair for volume and bend (for rolls or a pompadour), you would use an on-base or an over-directed base curl.

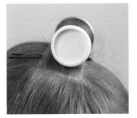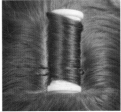

On base.

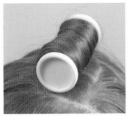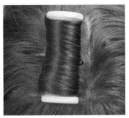

Over directed.

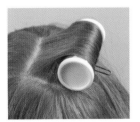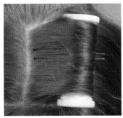

Off base.

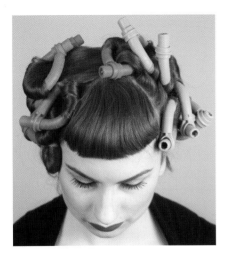

Right set on base; left off base.

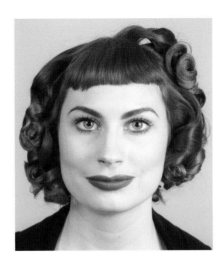

Difference in volume.

A 1940s SILHOUETTE

To create a typical 1940s silhouette of smooth crown and curled base, roll the lower half of the head on base and the top of the head off base, with a gap of around 5cm/2in between the sticks and the scalp. This will create a halo-like effect of curls.

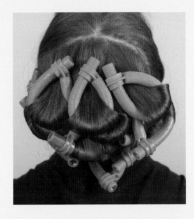

Top half of head set off base.

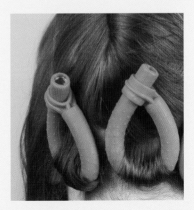

Lower half of head set on base.

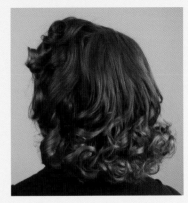

The classic U-shaped style.

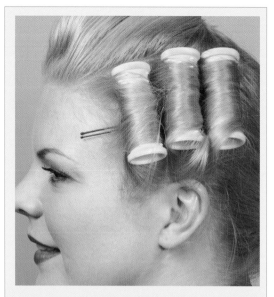

Rollers placed vertically.

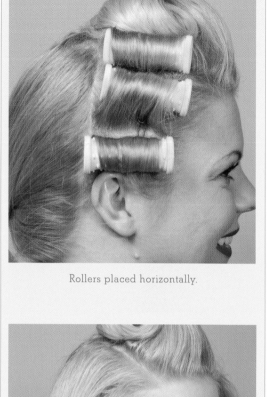

Rollers placed horizontally.

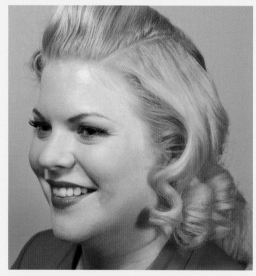

Produce ringlet curls.

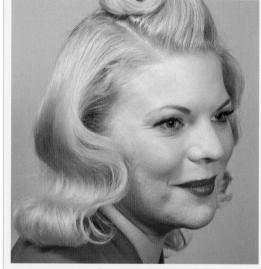

Produce a wave.

Curl Direction

The direction in which a curl is set will control the outcome of a set and how it sits. Whether you are using a hot or wet set, rollers or pin curls, the principle is the same. Curls all set in the same direction will create a smooth curl with all of the hair falling together (this is perfect for the Pageboy set). Curls that are set in alternating directions produce a wave as the curls sit in opposing directions and create ridges in the hair.

Rollers set vertically will produce a ringlet curl, which is perfect for creating ringlets and fluff.

Here, we can see an example of the same roller set in different directions.

Using End Papers

If the ends of the hair are not rolled

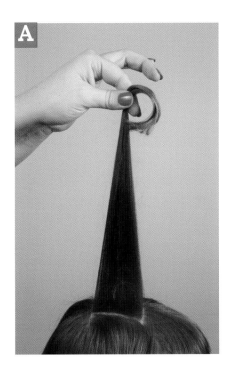

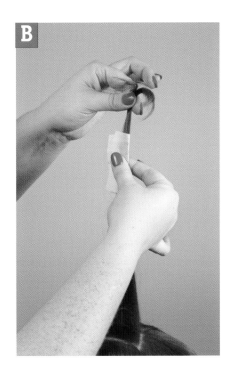

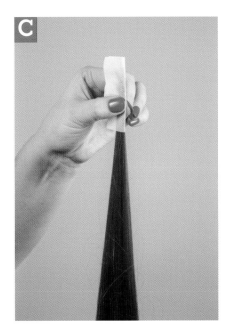

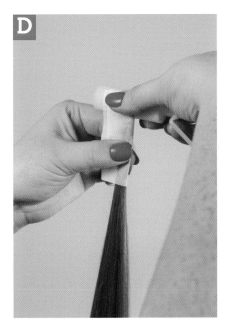

neatly, your set will be messy and frizzy. If you have problems tucking in the ends, try using end papers to hold together the loose ends of the hair. This makes it easier to curl the ends around the rollers, hot sticks and other curling techniques, wet or dry.

Directions

1. Take the section of hair. (A)
2. Fold the paper over the hair a few centimetres from the ends. (B)
3. Pull the paper upwards, holding the ends of the hair together. (C)
4. Roll the hair as normal. (D)

Creating Curls with Heat

Heat is a very popular method of curling hair. For most types of hair, heat will produce an attractive curl for a few hours, providing the temperature is high enough and the heat source is applied correctly. If your hair is naturally curly/wavy, you can even get a few days out of a hot set. For people with naturally very straight, silky hair, it can be tricky to achieve a satisfactory result as the curls will quickly drop and also the set does not have the strength to be moulded vigorously. There are some tricks that can be used to overcome this,

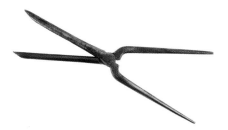

Vintage curling tongs

but if you hair will not take to heat, you may want to move on to wet setting.

Just as a wet set must dry to have the desired effect, a hot set must cool completely. If you have hair that is resistant to curling, try leaving the set for as long as possible before brushing out. This will also help to prolong the life of the curl. For example, leaving a hot pin curl set (created with a tong) overnight will produce a much stronger set than one left for just an hour.

Hot Rollers

Rollers produce soft curls with moderate holding power. Consequently, for many they are not the best tools for creating the structured and defined waves of the 1940s and you may find other methods more effective. Nevertheless, if you have hair with a good natural curl or that is chemically treated with bleach, you may find you can achieve a sufficient curl this way. Using a roller with a very small width will help create a more defined curl, but if your hair is naturally straight and stubborn, I would move straight to tongs or hot sticks to roll your set.

When set on base in the hair, large to medium rollers are very useful for creating bend and volume before attempting styles such as Victory Rolls, pompadours and other up-dos. Pre-curling makes these styles easier to execute.

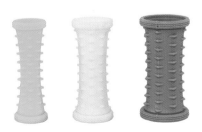

Hot rollers.

Directions

1. Take a section of hair the same width and length of the roller and mist the section with heat protector. (A)
2. Firmly tuck the ends of the hair around the roller. (B)

3. If you have problems tucking in the ends, you can use a tail comb to hold the ends securely as you start to roll. (C)
4. Roll the roller to the scalp, maintaining good tension on the hair. (D)

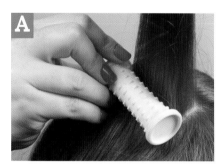

Hot rollers.

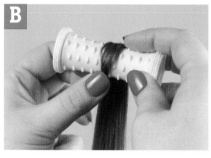

Tuck ends.

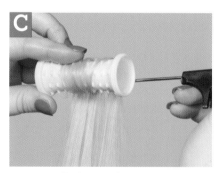

Tuck ends if needed.

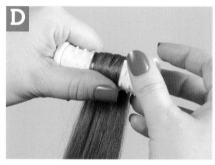

Roll to scalp.

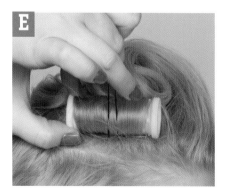

Use anchoring motion...

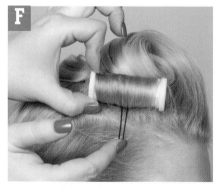

... with large hairpins to secure.

5. If needed, secure with roller clips or large hairpins, using an anchoring motion. (E,F)
6. Allow the set to cool completely for as long as possible.

Hot Sticks

Hot sticks are one of the best hot tools for creating a 1940s look. They are very similar in size to your finger, so they are perfect for emulating the effect of a traditional wet pin curl set (a curl formed around your finger and pinned flat to the scalp). Once again, attention must be paid to the ends when setting, using end papers if necessary.

The springy curls can be separated to produce a fluffy curl or brushed into smooth waves. Hot sticks also have the benefit of heating and cooling quickly, so they are effective when you are in a hurry. Furthermore, they are great for giving the illusion of thickness in fine hair.

Directions

1. Remove all tangles from the hair.
2. Divide the hair into horizontal

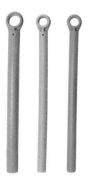

Hot sticks.

sections around the width of the stick. If your hair curls well, take a slightly larger section, and a smaller section if it is difficult to curl. The section can be wider horizontally than the stick, making a tube. Wrap the hair around the stick, ensuring the ends are tucked neatly. (A, B)

3. Roll the stick to the scalp and tuck the end inside the loop to secure. (C,D)
4. Leave the hot sticks to cool completely for as long as possible.

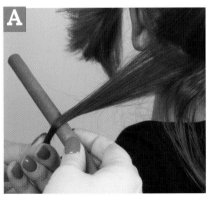

Wrap around stick.

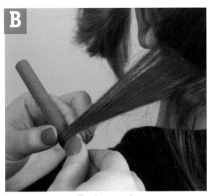

Tuck in end.

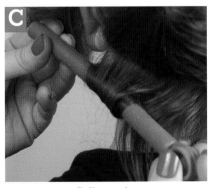

Roll to scalp.

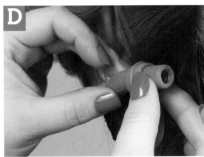

Secure.

Curling Tongs

Curling tongs come in many sizes and are great for creating smooth, robust curls. To achieve the strongest set, curl the hair to create a tube, then pin with curl clips and leave to cool completely before brushing out.

When curling, always start from the middle of the hair rather than the ends. The ends of your hair are fragile and less robust than the roots; they will curl more quickly but need protection from excess heat to avoid breakage and damage. Therefore, start curling towards the root area, working the ends into the tong.

If you have colour-treated or fragile hair, use a good-quality heat protector and keep the tongs on a lower hot setting.

Directions

1. Ensure the hair is free from tangles.
2. Protect the hair with a thermal spray.
3. Open the shell of the tongs and insert halfway down the shaft of the hair. (A)
4. Close the shell and wrap the hair around the tong while holding the ends of the hair. (B)
5. Still holding the hair with your fingertips, continuously rotate the tongs, gently opening and closing the shell of the tongs so that the ends of the hair are worked into the curl. (C)
6. Once all the hair is inside the tong,

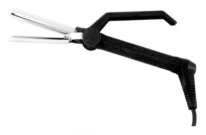
Curling tongs

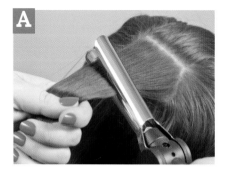

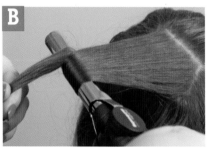

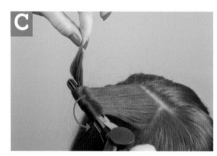

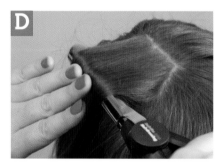

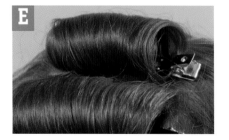

touch the hair to check it is warm throughout the curl. Once you are sure it is, release the shell and gently pull the tong from the hair, using your other hand to secure the curl. (D)
7. You will be left with an empty curl/tube. Clip the curl in place to cool completely before dressing out. (E)

This will produce a smooth, finished curl with the ends tucked neatly in the middle of the section.

TIP

Best for: Hair that is hard to curl; creating structured waves.

Avoid: Using tongs that are too hot on fragile, very chemically treated hair.

Always: Start the curl halfway down the hair shaft rather than at the ends. The ends of the hair are the most fragile and will curl the quickest, so work these into the curl after the middle and upper part of the section are sufficiently heated.

Make sure: You work the very ends of the tong into the hair or you will get hooked ends. Use a heat protector.

My hair is stubborn to curl: Use a smaller tong for a tighter curl. Try a mist of hairspray on the hair before you roll. DO NOT try this technique on fragile or very chemically treated hair as it can damage it.

Hot Pin Curls

Hot pin curls are created by tonging the hair, rolling the warm curl flat to the scalp and clipping it in place to cool. Read the instructions for pin curl direction in the 'Pin Curls' section as the same rules apply when setting hot pin curls.

This is the strongest set you can create with heat, with the added bonus of being able to leave it in overnight for even more staying power.

Directions

1. Take a section of hair the same width as the tong. (A)
2. Following the instructions above for using tongs, tong the section and remove the tongs from the hair. You

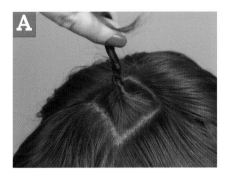

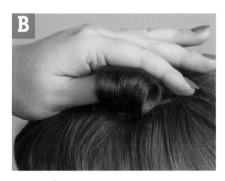

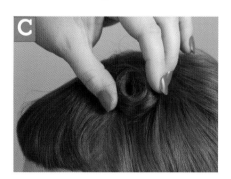

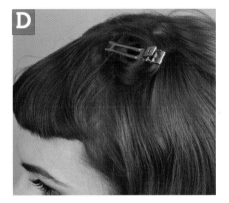

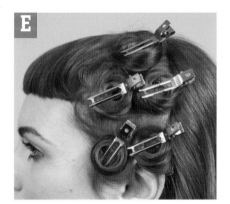

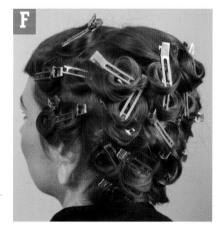

will be left with a small tube of hair. (B)

3. Flatten the tube, pushing together the two open ends of the curl and sit against the head in the desired direction (C). You can also keep the hair in an elevated curl (tube shape) which gives maximum volume, perfect for the crown area.
4. Clip into place with hairpins or pin curl clips. (D)
5. Continue around the head. (E,F)
6. Once all the curls are in place, mist with hairspray.
7. Leave the curls to cool and set for as long as possible, preferably overnight.

8. Protect with a net or scarf to avoid damaging the set while you sleep. (G)

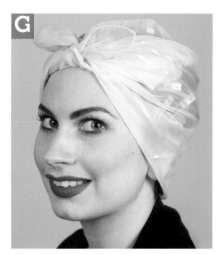

TIP

Best for: All hair types. This is the best heat method for hard to curl hair.

Avoid: Using tongs that are too hot on fragile, very chemically treated hair.

Use: A heat protector.

I have hair that is stubborn to curl: Try a mist of hairspray on the hair before you roll it, but DO NOT try this on fragile or very chemically treated hair, as it can damage it.

Wet Setting

The most popular and effective way of curling the hair in the 1940s and also today is with water and is known as a wet set.

A wet set is a method of curling the hair while it is wet/damp, using either pin curls, rollers or rags. The hair is left until completely dry and then brushed out in the desired style. This can either be done overnight or all day with the hair wrapped in a scarf or net, or a hood dryer can be used if speed is needed.

In addition to water, women in the 1940s would use a setting lotion. Using a setting lotion makes the hair more pliable and enables the curl to be held for longer.

A wet set is so effective as a result of the chemical process that takes place as the hair transitions from wet to dry. The water and tension on the hair causes the chemical bonds to break and reform as the hair dries, setting the hair in its new shape. Hair must be completely dry before brushing out the set or the chemical process will not work. This is why being caught in the rain without a bonnet or brolly can be truly disastrous for a lady's style!

Even today, with the multitude of heated implements on offer, a wet set is still the best way to produce an authentic vintage hairstyle. Wet sets have great staying power and are more malleable – perfect for all hair types and the best way to curl straight or stubborn hair. A well-maintained wet set can last for many days, which is far longer than a hot set for most people. Moreover, using water presents a far lower chance of damage compared with heating or perming.

Prepping the Hair for a Wet Set

To set the hair, you will need setting lotion and water. Some setting lotions do not need to be diluted with water, but

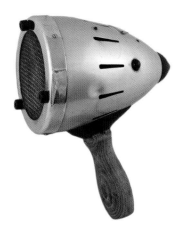

Vintage electric hair dryer.

the concept is the same as the hair is going from wet to dry. The correct way to apply this and the formulation used will depend on your hair type; therefore, you should experiment to discover what works best for you. Outlined below are three methods of prepping the hair.

METHOD 1
The first method is to set the hair directly after washing. Start by towel-drying the hair to remove a good amount of the moisture. Next, apply your chosen setting lotion throughout and set the hair.

This method works well for some, but if you have hair that dries quickly, you will need to mist some sections as you roll, otherwise the set may produce an uneven finish.

METHOD 2
Some people find that, even if they remove excess water by towel-drying, the hair does not get sufficiently dry, especially if it is very long and thick. In this case, you might want to try the spray

method. This works by wetting the hair as you go along. The precision of this method works well as you have more control over how wet the hair becomes, tailoring it to your hair thickness and the way it behaves. As mentioned previously, vintage styling involves trial and error. It is all about learning what works for your hair type.

If you are curling freshly washed hair, simply blast it dry with a hair dryer or wait for it to air dry if you do not wish to use heat. Once dry, brush through to remove any tangles from the hair. Mix the setting lotion in a spray bottle and mist the sections to be rolled one by one as you work around the head.

METHOD 3
Another approach is to mix the lotion and water in a bowl. Dip your fingers into the solution, smoothing it over each section as you roll up the hair. This is especially good for people with very thick hair or hair that takes an age to dry.

TIP **FOR THE PERFECT SET**

- When setting, the hair should be damp rather than wet to ensure the moisture is evenly applied through each section of hair. If the ends are not dampened sufficiently then the ends may become very frizzy when you brush them out.
- Make sure you ribbon each section of hair before you roll, creating tension in the hair.
- After the hair is set, it must be completely dry before you begin to dress it out. If it is not, it will not hold or withstand the brushing needed to shape into your chosen style.

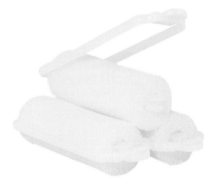

Sponge rollers.

Sponge Rollers

The sponge roller, when used correctly, is great for producing robust sets with lots of body. They are available in many different sizes ranging from very small to large, so pick the size relevant to the style you wish to create.

Directions

1. Prepare the hair for a wet set.
2. Wrap the damp hair around the roller, ensuring you tuck in the end neatly. (A)
3. Roll to scalp. (B)
4. Continue around the heads, making sure to tuck the bar of the roller underneath each time. (C)
5. Cover with a hairnet or scarf to protect your hair while you sleep.
6. Ensure your hair is completely dry before removing the rollers.

Always try to move the plastic bar to underneath the roller once in the hair, especially at the hairline, or you can get an indent in the hair after it dries. This can be clipped into place with a pin curl clip at the back of the roller if needed, to ensure it does not roll or flop forwards again.

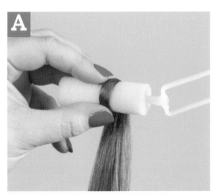

Tuck in end.

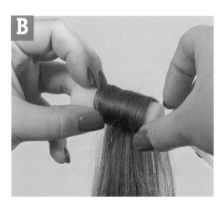

Roll to scalp and secure.

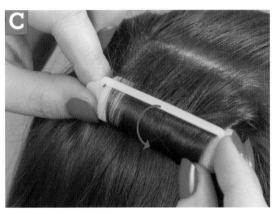

Tuck bar underneath.

 TIP

Best for: Straight hair that is hard to curl; creating waves.

Avoid: Very small rollers on naturally curly hair.

Never: Pull the hair too tightly around the roller, distorting the foam and creating a dent in the middle. This will distort the set and create frizz. Gently roll the hair around the roller so it retains its original shape.

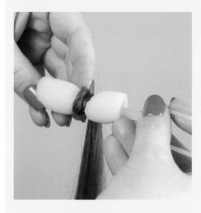

I can't tuck the ends in neatly: Try using end papers to hold the ends of the hair together as you roll.

My hair is so frizzy: Dampen the ends sufficiently before rolling. Use end papers to ensure the ends tuck smoothly around the roller. If your hair is very frizzy or naturally curly, you could try applying a small amount of natural oil, such as argan oil, to the ends before rolling.

My hair is very thick: You may find it hard to avoid indents from the plastic bar. If you get this problem, try smaller sections or move on to Velcro rollers.

The rollers keep falling out of my hair: Secure with pin curl clips while your set dries, sliding them into the middle of the roller, or with a large hairpin using a lever action.

Velcro Rollers

Velcro rollers are available in a variety of sizes and have stiff, grabbing teeth that secure the roller in the hair.

Be careful when using Velcro rollers as it is easy to get in a tangle. If you have very fine, delicate hair, you will probably be better off using a sponge roller or trying pin curls as an alternative. I also advise never trying to sleep in the hard Velcro rollers as the small prongs do not make for a comfy night's sleep. You can purchase Velcro rollers with a sponge inner, which are easier to sleep in but can still take some getting used to.

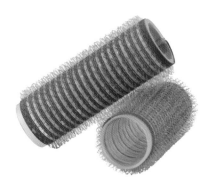

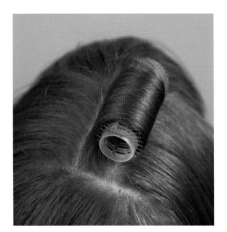

Velcro rollers.

Directions

1. Prep the hair for a wet set.
2. Section the hair so that it is no wider or thicker than the roller you have chosen.
3. Starting at the ends of the hair, tuck the ends neatly onto the roller and roll to the scalp, maintaining a good tension.

 TIP

Best for: Sets that require a lot of volume; thick hair or hair that takes a long time to dry, as lots of air can circulate around the set.

Avoid: Using on delicate or fragile hair.

My hair is so frizzy: Dampen the ends sufficiently before rolling. Use end papers to ensure the ends curl smoothly around the roller. If your hair is very frizzy and naturally curly, you could try applying a small amount of natural oil, such as argan oil, to the ends before rolling.

Rag Rollers

As the name suggests, these rollers are made of fabric and produce a strong and curly set. Leftover fabric is ripped into strips and used to roll up the hair into tight curls. The same technique was used with scraps of paper, such as old grocery bags, but I wouldn't recommend this as the paper could disintegrate in the hair. Attention must be paid to the ends of the hair when rolling for a smooth finish. Take around a finger's width of hair, or smaller pieces for tighter curls, bigger for larger curls. The tightness or looseness of your curl is

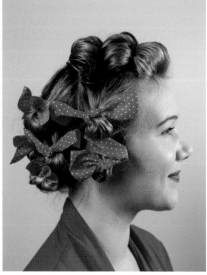

Rag rollers.

determined by the number of curls you roll and their thickness.

Rag curls can be easier to master than pin curls, as you can roll the hair in much bigger sections. However, be aware that the bigger the section, the longer it will take to dry. If you have very thick hair, the set will take longer to dry due to the lack of air circulating around it. Prep in exactly the same way as for a pincurl set.

Directions

1. Cut or rip your rags to around 5x13 centimetres (2x5 inches) long.
2. Prepare the hair for a wet set.
3. Divide the hair into sections of around 2.5cm/1in wide.
4. To create a large rag curl, wrap the hair around the rag and the width of one or two fingers. For a smaller curl, wrap the hair only around the fabric. (A,B)
5. Tuck in the ends and roll to the scalp. (C,D E)
6. Tie the ends to secure, and continue around the head. (F,G)
7. Leave the hair to dry completely before brushing out.

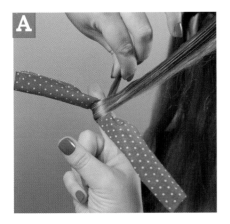

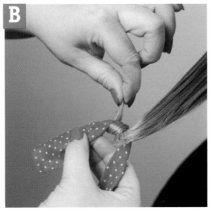

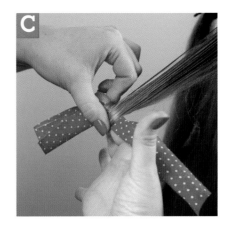

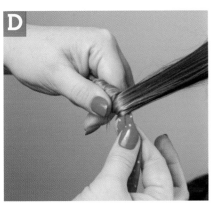

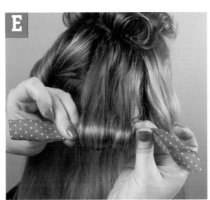

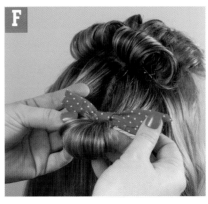

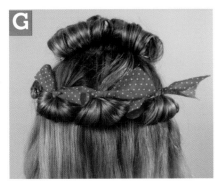

8. Finish the top crown section of this set with stand-up pin curls or use rag curls following the instructions above. Note that the curls will be very tight so you might want to roll the rag curls at the crown slightly off base on the front section.

9. A hood dryer can help with the drying process, as this method can be the longest to dry of all the wet sets.

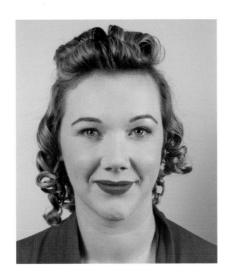

On the right is the effect of the rag curl wrapped around the fabric only, while the hair wrapped around a single finger is illustrated on the left. You can see the difference in tightness between the two.

Pin Curls

One of the most popular methods used for hairstyles in the 1940s was the wet pin curl set. A pin curl is the technique by which hair is divided into sections, formed around a finger, fingers or pin-curling device, and pinned or clipped to the head. The hair is left to dry completely and then brushed out.

Pin curls are perfect for creating an authentic look. Once your hair has been set in pin curls, it becomes more malleable and can stand up to vigorous brushing as you shape your hair into your desired style. Pin curl sets are also very long-lasting. The method gives the hair lots of bounce, and the staying power of the set means less hairspray is used, providing more natural movement.

A well-maintained pin curl set can last for at least two days for most hair types and up to four or five days for curly hair. Once the original set has dropped out, there is still some curl and texture in the hair; therefore, on the second or third day the hair is in a perfect state for styling into Victory Rolls, pompadours or other styles.

There are several technical aspects to setting pin curls that can be a little daunting for a beginner, but please do not be intimidated if you have not attempted pin curls before. The most important factor to remember is to prepare the hair correctly with water and setting lotion and ensure all the ends are neatly tucked. All the other skills can be added once you get the knack of rolling the pin curls.

If you are already a pin-curling pro, take a few minutes to refresh your knowledge of the techniques. The same principles of base direction, curl direction, tension and width of curl, as mentioned at the beginning of this chapter, all apply to pin curls.

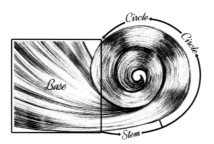
Anatomy of a pin curl.

ANATOMY OF A PIN CURL

The circle: This is the part of the pin curl that forms a complete circle, the curl. The size of the circle determines the width of the wave and its strength, with a smaller circle or pin curl having a tighter curl than a bigger one. For the styles presented in this book, pin curls are made with an open circle. This produces a smooth, even curl that is the same size throughout. A closed circle would mean the ends of the hair would have a tighter curl than the top, producing a fluffier curl.

The base: This is the stationary foundation of the curl. This can be sectioned in different shapes; this book uses triangular, square and rectangular bases:

- **Triangular base:** used when curling the hairline to avoid any gaps and breaks in the finished hairstyle.
- **Square base:** this is the most common base. It is used for elevated and flat pin curls. It is typically 2.5cm/1in wide.
- **Rectangular base:** used on elevated pin curl sets as they can be set in wider sections, replacing 2–4 pin curls. When used at the side-front hairline, they create a smooth, up-swept effect.

The stem: This is the section of the pin curl between the base and the first arc of the circle. The stem can be different lengths and gives the curl its direction

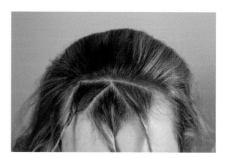
Triangular base.

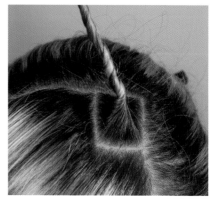
Square base.

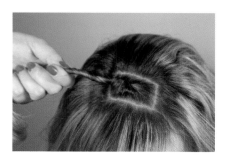
Rectangular base.

and movement. The direction in which the curl and stem are placed will determine the finished style.

PIN CURL BASE PLACEMENT

The way in which the curl or circle is pinned to the base will ultimately determine the volume and final outcome of the style:

No Stem Curl: This is placed directly on the base of the curl and produces a tight, firm, long-lasting curl. This is the

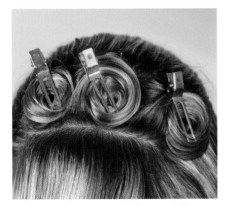

Left to right: no stem, half stem, full stem.

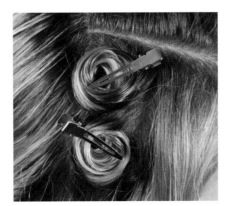

Reverse and forward curl.

hardest pin curl to master as it is tricky to get the curl exactly on base without distorting and squashing it.

Half/Small Stem: The curl is placed half off the base. The hair retains its volume and produces an even curl throughout the hair. Half-off-base curls have been used for most of the styles detailed in this book as they produce a smooth and workable curl.

Full/Large Stem: This curl is placed completely off base. The length of the stem means that minimum volume is produced, as the section of hair near the roots is straight. Use it for styles where you want minimum body with curl just at the ends of the hair.

PIN CURL DIRECTION
Pin curls are set in two main directions: Forwards (rolling towards the face) and Reverse (away from the face).

They are also set in either clockwise or counterclockwise directions. For example, a pin curl on the left side of the head rolling forwards to the face would be a clockwise curl, whilst a pin curl rolling towards the face on the right side would be a counterclockwise curl.

The way in which the curl/stem is directed affects the final style:

- When the curl is directed forward, the hair will style towards the face.
- When the curl is directed backward, the hair will style away from the face.
- When the curl is directed upward, the hair will style in an upward flip.
- When the curl is directed downward the hair will flip under.

CREATING WAVES
Set the pin curls in alternate rows of forward and reverse curls. This is known as a skip wave, as the opposing directions of the rows produce ridges in the hair.

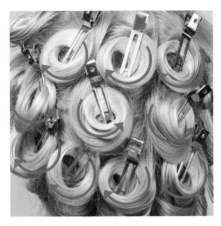

Skip wave.

CREATING CURLS
If the pin curls are all directed the same way, you can create more of a smooth wave or barrel curl, with the curls falling together. These curls can also be brushed into defined ringlet curls or fluff curls.

PIVOT POINT
The pivot point is the angle at which you roll the pin curl to the head. A correct pivot point is created by rolling the curl at a diagonal to the base. This means that it sits perfectly on the base, not distorting the shape. If you roll the curl from directly underneath or above the base, it will create curls that stick out at funny angles and will not create a smooth finish.

Take a look at these pin curls and note the diagonal angle at which they are

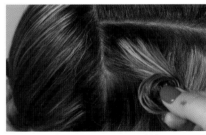

Correct pivot point (A).

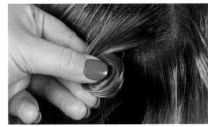

Correct pivot point (B).

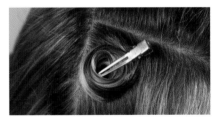

Curl sitting correctly.

rolled towards the scalp, thereby allowing them to sit neatly.

PIN CURL SIZES
Pin curls are formed mostly around the fingers; therefore, small, medium and large pin curls are easy to measure in terms of the width of one, two or three fingers.

Try to maintain the same size and shape of pin curl and base to ensure an even set.

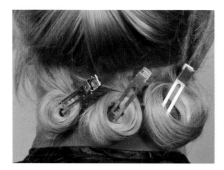
Different pin curl sizes.

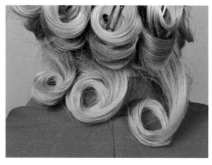
Different sizes of curl.

KIT LIST
Brush
Comb
Hairpins/Curl Clips
Hairnet/Scarf
Setting Lotion
Spray Bottle (optional)
Hood or Bonnet Dryer (optional)

PIN CURL TUTORIALS

Method 1
This is the most common method, which involves forming the curl around your finger or pin-curling device.

1. Prep the hair for a wet set.
2. Section the hair.
3. Ribbon the section.
4. Place your finger (or fingers depending on desired curl size) a centimetre or two from the end of the hair and wrap the hair around your finger until you reach the end of the hair. (A)
5. Tuck in the end, holding it securely in place with your thumb. (B)
6. Carefully pull your finger from the curl and you will be left with a neat curl with a clear centre. (C,D)
7. Roll the curl to the scalp with your fingertips, making sure not to twist or distort it and ensuring the end is tucked neatly. (E)
8. Clip the curl to the scalp with pin curl clips or hairpins. Pinning through the 'stem' keeps the curl secure. (F)
9. If you are sleeping on the curls, protect them with a slumber net or scarf (nets are better for thick hair as they allow more air to circulate the set and aid drying).

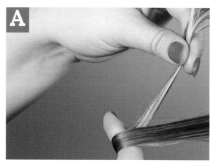
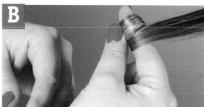
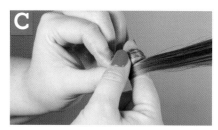
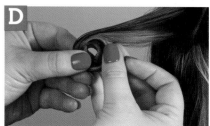
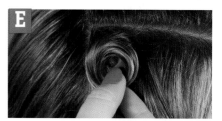
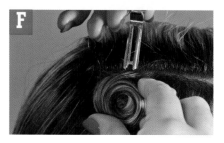

Method 2

This involves curling the hair right next to the scalp. This method takes some practice to ensure no ends are left sticking out. Do not pull the curl too tightly while rolling, as it will be difficult to pull the curl off your finger.

1. Prep the hair for a wet set.
2. Part a section.
3. Ribbon the hair.
4. Place your index finger against the scalp at the base of the section. Note that the finger is not placed in the centre of the section as the curl will be distorted and will not brush out well. (A)
5. Lift your finger slightly from the head, creating enough space for the hair to be wrapped around it. Wrap until you reach the end of the hair, taking care not to twist the strand. (B)
6. Tuck in the end, making sure it is not sticking out. (C)
7. Carefully remove your finger from the curl. (D,E)
8. Pin to the scalp. (F)
9. Allow the hair to dry completely before you begin to brush out.
10. If you are sleeping on the curls, protect them with a slumber net or scarf (nets are better for thick hair as they allow more air to circulate and aid drying).

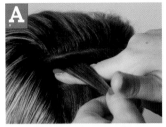
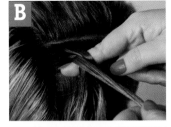
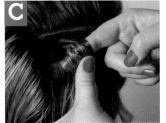
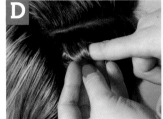
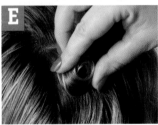
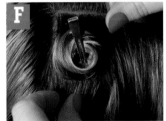

Method 3

1. Part a section.
2. Ribbon the section.
3. Form the pin curl at the very end of the hair. (A,B)
4. Roll to the scalp, keeping the ends tucked in neatly. (C,D)
5. Pin to the scalp.
6. Allow the hair to dry completely before you begin to brush out.
7. If you are sleeping on the curls, protect them with a slumber net or scarf (nets are better for thick hair as they allow more air to circulate and aid drying).
8. Allow the hair to dry completely before you begin to brush out.
9. If you are sleeping on the curls, protect them with a slumber net or scarf (nets are better for thick hair as they allow more air to circulate and aid drying).

Troubleshooting tips for pin curls are given below in the 'Elevated pin curl section'.

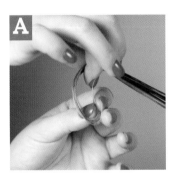
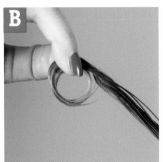
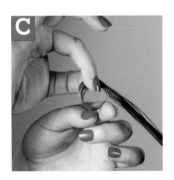
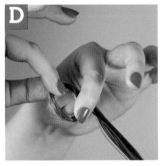

ELEVATED PIN CURLS

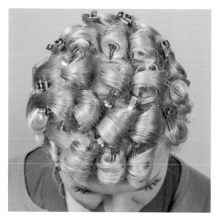

Elevated pin curls are those that stand up from the scalp. They help create volume and are typically used on the crown, but can be used all over the head. Also known as stand-up pin curls, they provide more lift at the base of the curl than a flat pin curl.

Elevated pin curls can be rolled on base or off base depending on the amount of volume you prefer.

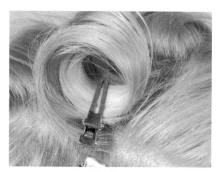

On base.

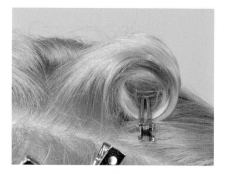

Off base.

Directions

1. When curling at the hairline, use a triangular base to avoid obvious partings or gaps when the hair is dry.
2. Ribbon the hair, removing tangles and creating a nice tension.
3. Wrap the hair around your finger or fingers and tuck the end in securely. (A,B)
4. Roll to the scalp. (C,D)
5. Fix the curl with a single-pronged curl clip, as these are easier to slide into the hair. (E)
6. If you are sleeping on stand-up pin curls all over the head, then try to dry them partially with a dryer before sleeping to avoid squashing the shape. If the curls are only on top of the head, it is easier to keep the shape.
7. A hairnet is useful to protect the stand-up pin curls as you sleep.

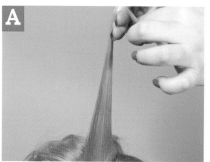

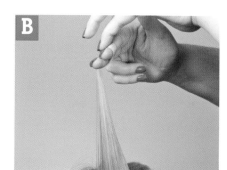

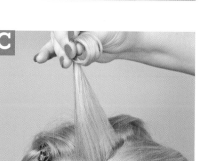

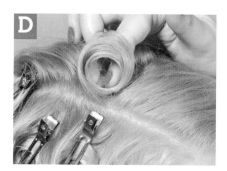

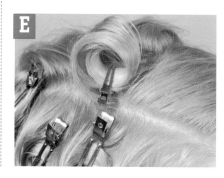

Best for: All hair types but especially difficult to curl tresses; an authentic 1940s look.

Avoid: Very small pin curls on naturally curly and thick hair.

Make sure: You do not twist the hair when creating the pin curls or you will end up with a lot of frizz and not a great finish.

Do not: Squash the pin curls when pinning them as this will distort them. Pin through the stem to secure the curl easily.

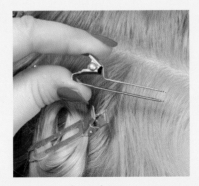

Large hinge.

For thick hair: Use pins with an extra-large hinge to avoid squashing the hair.

The pins/clips make dents in my hair: This may be an issue if you have thick hair. Try changing methods if this happens, as some people find curl clips work for them while hairpins produce dents, and vice versa. As with all hair techniques, it is not a 'one size fits all' method; experiment to see which method works best for you. Make sure you are using clips without indents on them as they may imprint.

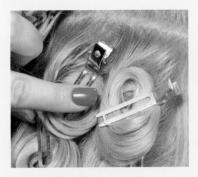

Squashed pin curl.

I cannot get the ends to tuck into my pin curls: This is particularly hard on naturally straight hair and also tricky when you are just starting out with pin curls. To get used to the technique of tucking in the ends of the hair, try it the evening/day after a roller/tong or hot stick set when you have some bend in the end of the hair. This will help you get used to the motion and will help next time you try pin-curling from wet, straight hair.
You can also try using end papers. Fold the paper in half and tuck the hair into the fold. Wrap the paper around the end of the hair, so it is the same thickness as the rest, and roll as you would a normal pin curl.
Keeping the ends sufficiently damp will help gather them together when rolling into pin curls.

Even pin curls won't hold in my hair: Ensure the set is completely dry before brushing out the hair. For extra staying power, spray an even layer of firm-hold hairspray over the hair one hour before removing the clips. Try using a smaller pin curl to obtain more hold or using a small amount of firm-hold gel on your hair before setting.

The clips get hot against my skin under the dryer: Try placing a tissue or piece of cotton between your skin and the clips.

I don't have time for a wet set, but heat isn't effective: Try using a mousse to set the hair. This will dry much more quickly, but be careful not to overdo the mousse as it can become sticky and render the hair somewhat crispy.

Avoid frizz: By ensuring the ends of the pin curl are sufficiently damp; by getting the ends of your hair trimmed regularly.

PIN-CURLING ACCESSORIES

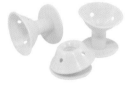

Pin curl rollers.

Even in the 1940s, all sorts of gadgets were being invented to make hairstyling easier. The Curl Master hair-winding rod from Curly Lox Products was exactly the same shape as a traditional dolly peg, but it was double-ended with one small dolly peg and one large peg. Due to the similarity in design to a dolly peg, they can be used to create pin curls and keep the ends neat.

Dolly Peg Curls

These make small, uniform pin curls.

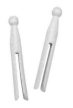

Directions

1. Ribbon the hair.
2. Take a section of hair and angle in the direction you wish the curl to roll.
3. Insert your hair into the dolly peg, a few centimetres from the ends. (A)
4. Slide down to the end until you are holding just the tip of the hair. (B)
5. Hold the ends securely with your thumb and tuck them in, starting to roll the peg. (C)
6. Roll the hair around the peg towards the scalp, tucking in flyaway hairs as you go. (D)
7. Rest the peg on the scalp. Secure the curl with a finger whilst you slide out the peg. (E,F)
8. Secure the curl with a curl clip. (G)
9. Leave the hair to dry thoroughly before brushing out.

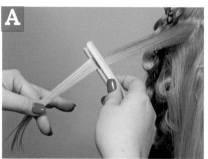

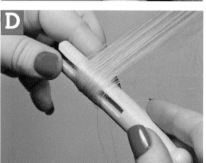

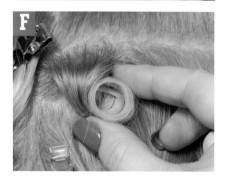

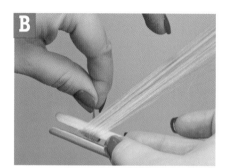

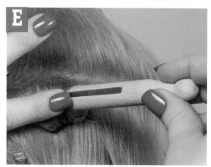

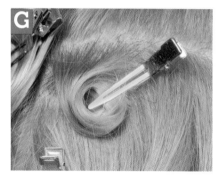

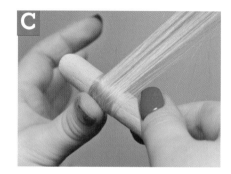

TIP

Do not: place the curl directly in the centre of the base as it will become distorted (see the section on pin curl base placement for more information).

Do not: pull the hair too tightly around the dolly peg or it will be hard to slide out. If you still cannot remove the peg, try rubbing it with a bit of argan oil to allow the hair to slide off more easily.

I don't have a dolly peg: Try forming the pin curl around an object, such as a mascara tube, and rolling the hair to the scalp then pinning into place.

Creating Curls with Extensions

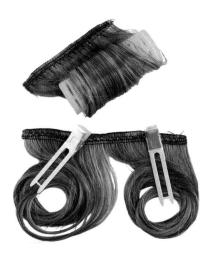

Extension wefts.

When selecting extensions, ensure you get the best colour match for your hair. Take your extensions to your hairdresser and ask him or her to clip them in and cut them, blending them with your own hair to the length you desire, adding some layers. Remember, once they are curled they will spring up a centimetre or two depending on the tightness of the curl. Try and purchase extensions with silicone strips on the clips; this helps them sit firmly in the hair without needing to add back-combing to the roots.

When curling real hair extensions you can use heat (tongs work well) or water, although I find water produces a better result. The best option for curling extensions with water is with pin curls or Velcro rollers. Set the curl in the extensions before you clip them to the head.

Finger Waves

Finger waves are created by using a comb and fingers to shape and direct wet hair into an S formation. This is then left to dry fully and brushed out.

Finger waves were extremely popular in the 1920s and 1930s. By the 1940s the full head of finger waves had become unfashionable, but partial waves on the crown or side of the head remained popular. The wave was combed in and then any remaining ends were rolled into pin curls. Alternatively, the waves were created with pin curls, producing the waved look but with greater volume. Waves could be wide or narrow and with or without defined ridges.

RIDGE WAVE

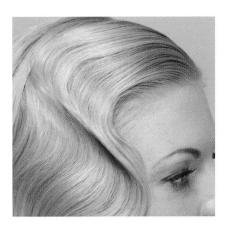

Ridge wave

This wave has prominent ridges with lots of definition.

Directions

1. Make sure the section to be waved is nice and wet with lots of setting lotion or a small amount of gel applied evenly throughout. (A)
2. Firmly comb the hair back diagonally from the face. Make sure the teeth of the comb connect with the scalp. (B)
3. Place your index finger securely on the scalp. (C)
4. Comb the hair in the opposite direction to the first section, at a diagonal. (D)
5. Insert the teeth of the comb into the hair around 1 cm (in) below your index finger and push upwards in the opposite direction to the way the hair was combed. You will see that a ridge has been created. (E)
6. Lift your index finger and move it underneath the ridge, pinching it together slightly. Ensure you keep firm pressure on the head with your middle finger, sliding it downwards to the previous position of your index finger. (F)
7. Comb the hair diagonally, in the opposite direction to the first comb. (G)
8. Once again, work your fingers down the hair with your middle finger being replaced by your ring finger, always keeping pressure on the hair. This will leave your middle finger holding the wave created in the hair. Comb the hair in the opposite direction, creating a curve in the hair. (H)
9. Insert the comb 1 cm (in) from the middle finger and push up again to create a ridge. (I)
10. Continue moving your fingers down the hair to create as many ridges as you desire.
11. Use long duck-billed clips to hold the ridges in place. (J)
12. Curl any loose ends into pin curls.
13. Allow to dry completely before brushing out.

> **TIP**
>
> **Do not:** try to increase the height of the ridge by lifting it up with the fingers. This will remove and distort the ridge formation off its base.
>
> **My hair is very thick:** Duck-billed clips with teeth will help secure the hair.

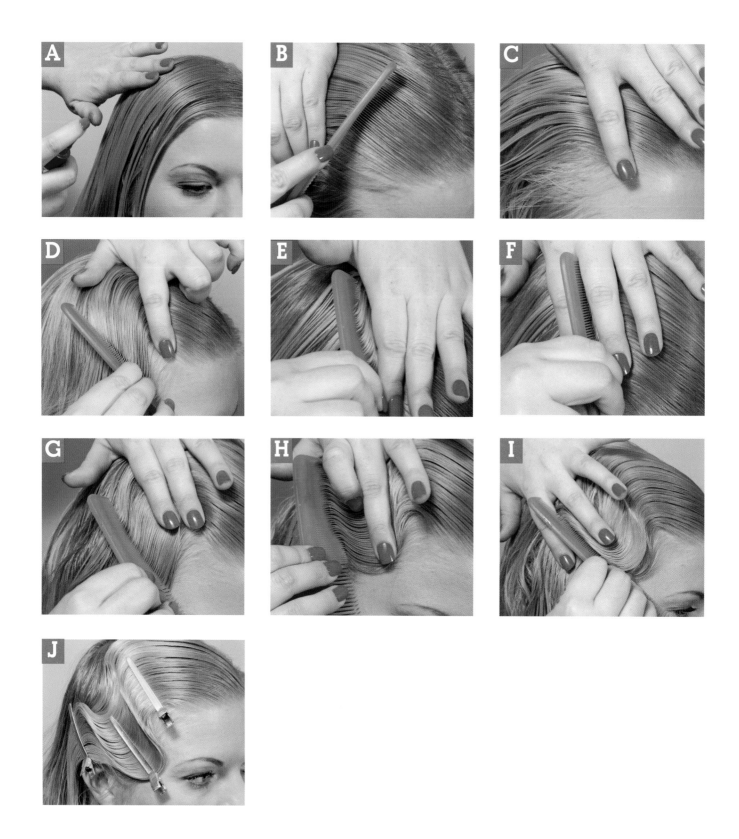

SHADOW WAVE

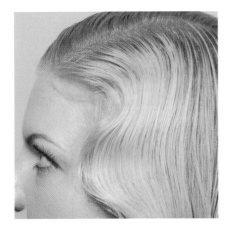

Shadow wave

This is a very soft wave with no ridges.

Directions

1. Make sure the section to be waved is nice and wet with lots of setting lotion or a small amount of gel applied evenly throughout. (A)
2. Firmly comb the hair back diagonally from the face. Make sure the teeth of the comb connect with the scalp. (B)
3. Place your index finger securely on the scalp. (C)
4. Comb the hair in the opposite direction to the first section, at a diagonal. (D)
5. Move your index finger downwards, putting pressure on the new wave in the hair. Use a duck-billed clip to secure the first wave in place. Firmly comb the hair in the opposite direction, making contact with the scalp. (E)
6. A wave has been created. (F)
7. Secure the hair with clips as you go, creating as many waves as you would like. (G)
8. Allow the hair to dry completely before brushing out.

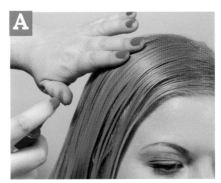

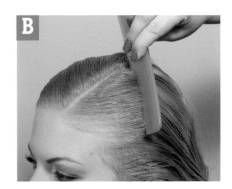

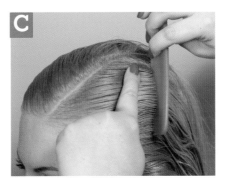

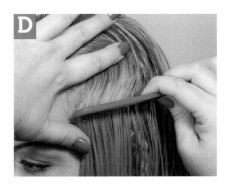

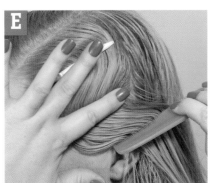

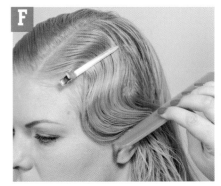

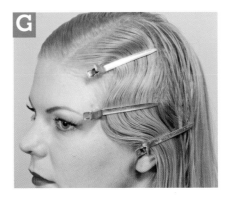

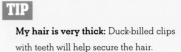

My hair is very thick: Duck-billed clips with teeth will help secure the hair.

Victory Rolls

The Victory Roll is a classic, tunnel-shaped curl that is closed and conical inside, and usually sits on top of the head. This style was adopted in the 1940s by working women and Hollywood starlets alike, namely Betty Grable, Veronica Lake and Rita Hayworth. Whether you were a film star or a factory worker, this quintessential 1940s style was immensely popular and worn day and night. This section outlines the style in detail and provides plenty of tips so that you can master it yourself.

When creating Victory Rolls, you can either start with straight hair or it can be pre-curled. For most people, especially those new to vintage hairstyling, there are real benefits to prepping the hair beforehand. With particularly straight or silky hair, pre-curling the hair bends it in the desired direction and rough shape, which makes the hair easier to manipulate.

If you have very fine hair and creating volume is a struggle, pre-setting the hair with rollers, hot sticks or large curls will give extra body to the hair and make the creation of the roll easier. Ensure you set the hair on base or with stand-up pin curls to give the hair as much volume as possible. Pre-setting can also help

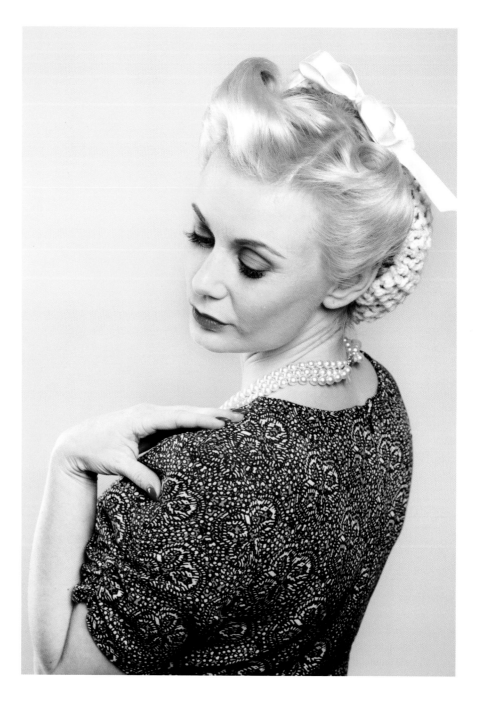

KIT LIST

Tail comb
Bristle brush
Sectioning clips
Hairpins
Kirby grips
Hairspray
Pomade
Dry shampoo (optional)
Curling device or flat irons (optional)

smooth out the texture of naturally curly hair; tongs are especially good for this as they create tension on the hair. Another technique is to go around the hairline with flat irons to remove kinks and frizz, producing a smoother roll.

As with many vintage styles, having hair that has not been washed for 24–48 hours will make life a lot easier; the hair will be less slippery and more malleable. If you are worried about greasy roots, use some dry shampoo.

I do not want to back-brush/comb my hair: This is still possible, but ensure you attempt the style on hair that has not been washed for at least 24–48 hours and avoid using slippery serums.

- Add a good amount of back-combing spray or powder to the hair, paying particular attention to the roots.
- Hold the hair at the desired angle for the roll and spray with hairspray, gently smoothing the top layer.
- Roll and secure the hair, remembering the structure will be more delicate without the benefit of back-brushing.
- Mist with a generous amount of hairspray.

I have too much hair to handle: Try rolling the hair into a series of smaller rolls, rather than two large rolls, while you get used to the technique.

I cannot get even rolls: I am a fan of asymmetrical styles, but the trick is doing them deliberately. Go for one large and one small roll on either side of the head. Not only easier, this option can be much more flattering.

How do I prolong my style? Sleep with your rolls wrapped in a hairnet or scarf. To neaten any flyaway hairs the next day, apply hairspray and smooth the top layer very gently with a brush or comb. You can also spray your hand and smooth this against the roll to neaten any rogue hairs. If you have very fine hair, your rolls may become flat overnight. Use the end of a tail comb to gently coax them away from the head by inserting the pointed end into the roll.

Victory Rolls don't suit me: Try experimenting with different partings and placements. Try adjusting the angles of the rolls and make them higher or flatter. Perhaps several small rolls will be more flattering than two big rolls. Try placing them further back on the head or moving them closer together or further apart. Also, try changing the angles from forwards to upwards facing.

My Victory Rolls look like horns/ears: Make sure you back-brush enough at the roots. If you concentrate only on the lengths, rather than the roots, the volume will all be at the top, which may result in a horned look. Two forward-facing, even rolls with a gap in between can occasionally resemble Mickey Mouse ears! To remedy this, make the rolls meet in the middle. They can have a roll or pomp in the middle to separate them. Alternatively, make sure that the roots of the roll have a lot of volume so you don't have two big rolls with a flat area in the middle.

This can be a particular problem for very long, fine hair. This type of hair is wound around so many times that it creates a lot of volume in the roll. Try creating more rolls or a diagonal parting and, again, ensure the roots are well back-brushed.

My hair is so fine, I can't get enough volume: Try a good application of dry shampoo or back-combing powder to the roots to build volume and make the hair stand out from the side of the head.

If you are creating a Victory Roll at the front with a curled back, try extension wefts at the back to build volume. This means you can take much larger sections at the front of the head for the rolls, enabling you to bulk them out. Back comb the hair in many thin sections, making sure you get lots of volume at the roots.

How do I remove the back-combing? Remove the back-combing gently while your hair is dry (wet hair is more prone to breakage). Use a specific detangling brush, as its flexible bristles will smooth the hair without causing any damage. For stubborn back-combing, put a small amount of conditioner on dry hair to help tease out knots.

For a round face: Make sure the Victory Rolls do not have too much volume at the sides or are rolled too loosely as this will widen your face. You want to aim for more volume and height at the top and flatter sides.

For a long face: Ensure you have volume at the sides and not too much on top to avoid elongating your face.

For a large forehead: Try Victory Rolls with a rolled fringe.

I have a fringe: You can still have Victory Rolls. You can either curl the fringe and work it into the rolls or keep your fringe down. To give it a more period look, I would advise curling it under slightly with straighteners or flipping under the outer corners of the fringe, Bettie Page-style.

Directions

1. Section the hair from ear to ear. (A)
2. If your hair is slippery, you could use a dry shampoo or back-combing powder to create texture.
3. Back-combing or back-brushing creates volume and texture, making the hair easier to roll and pin. Back-brush the hair in even, horizontal sections (about three), taking care to ensure you back-brush the roots (B,C). This will ensure the rolls look even. Add a mist of hairspray to each section. Do not back-brush your hair harshly; you are simply fluffing the hair to give it texture and volume. Using a bristle brush is far gentler on the hair.
4. Mist the hair with hairspray. (D)
5. Rub pomade through your fingertips to tame flyaway hairs and help with control as you work the hair into shape. (E)
6. Hold the hair out from the head at the angle where the roll will sit. Once in position, spray the section with hairspray and use a brush to gently smooth the very top layer of hair on the roll. Take care not to remove all the back-brushing (F,G). Mist the very ends with spray; this will make them easier to roll and secure in position. Pulling the hair further out from the head rather than straight and up helps create volume throughout the sides; pulling the hair upwards will create volume on top and give flatter sides.
7. Place your fingers on top of the hair, halfway up the length. Wrap the hair around your finger (or fingers), keeping the hair taut. (H) Some people like to start at the end but I think a mid-point is better as you have more control over the angle you are rolling as you are closer to the head.

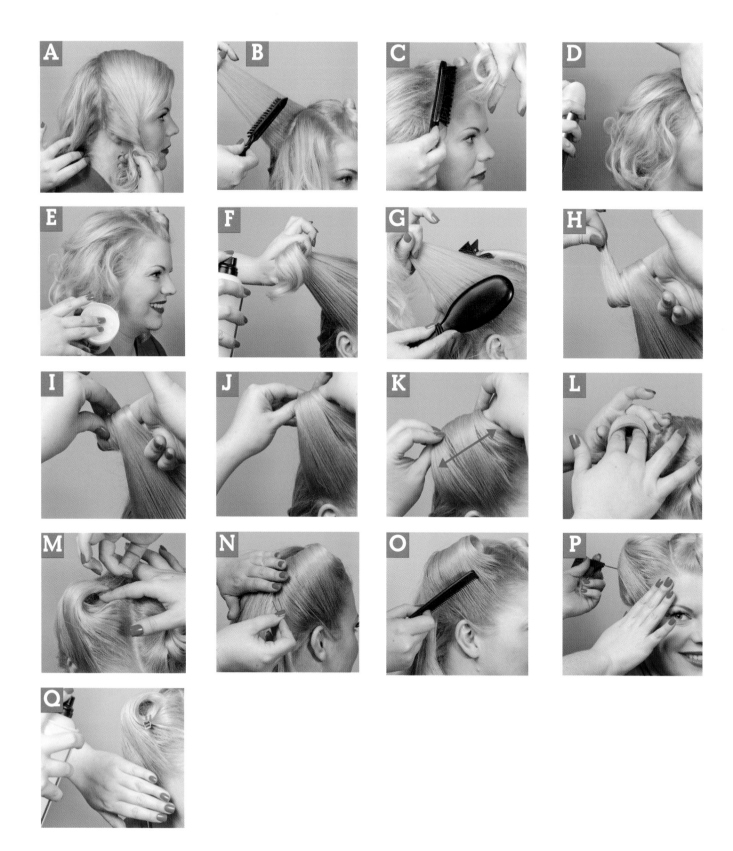

8. Tuck the end under your thumb and carefully pull your fingers out of the hair so you are left with a tube.(I)

9. Using both hands, continue rolling the tube towards the scalp, spreading it slightly as you go and lengthening the tube. Make sure you do not let go of the hair at this point. (J,K)

10. Gently sit the roll against the scalp. At this point you can make any adjustments to the shape with your fingertips. (L)

11. Holding the roll securely, carefully slide a Kirby grip into the top edge of the roll until it is hidden. (M)

12. Add more Kirby grips until the roll feels secure.

13. Gently push the roll down and back with one hand, so the back of the roll sits flat against the head, (N) and use hairpins secure it in place. Hairpins are less likely to distort the shape of the roll as they glide more smoothly than Kirby grips and effectively anchor the back of the roll to the head.

14. Spray the roll with hairspray and gently smooth the top with a brush or comb. You are not brushing into the hair; you are just gently sweeping over the surface to smooth the hair. (O)

15. Use your fingers and hairspray to smooth any flyaway hairs at the hairline or on the rolls.

16. Use a tail comb to make any adjustments to the rolls. (P)

17. Curl clips can also be used to make any final adjustments to the shape. (Q)

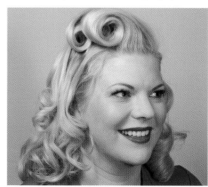

Victory Rolls can be rolled in various sizes and directions.

Barrel Rolls

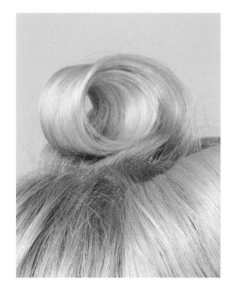

KIT LIST

Tail comb

Bristle brush

Sectioning clips

Hairpins

Kirby grips

Hairspray

Pomade

Dry shampoo (optional)

Barrel Rolls are created exactly the same way as Victory Rolls, but instead of the rolls being cone-shaped they are tube-shaped. Often, you can see right through the tunnel you create. Barrel rolls are used in multiple ways. They are the basis of a smooth roll at the nape of the neck or can sit together in multiples, creating interesting curl detail.

Directions

1. Take the section you wish to roll. This may be one large section or multiple smaller sections.

2. Divide the section into horizontal slices and add back-brushing throughout. (A)

3. Hold the hair from the head in the direction you wish to roll it, laying it flat over your hand. Mist with hairspray and gently smooth the top layer of hair, taking care not to disturb the teasing underneath. (B)

4. Depending on the desired thickness of the roll, take one or a few fingers and wrap the hair around the fingers, starting midway down the section of hair. (C)

5. Tuck the ends of the hair under your thumb and gently remove your fingers, leaving an empty tube. (D)

6. Gently grip the two ends of the tube

TIP

My hair is really fine: Use a back-combing powder or dry shampoo to add bulk and volume.

My hair is still too slippery to roll: Try using dry shampoo or a back-combing powder prior to rolling. Mist the ends with hairspray before you roll. Make sure your hair has not been washed for 24–48 hours.

I do not want to back-brush/comb my hair: This is still possible, but ensure you attempt the style on hair that has not been washed for at least 24–48 hours and avoid using slippery serums.

• Add a generous amount of back-combing spray or powder to hair, concentrating on the roots.

• Hold the hair at the desired angle for the roll and spray with hairspray, gently smoothing the top layer.

• Roll and secure the roll, remembering it will be more delicate without back-brushing.

• Mist with a good amount of hairspray.

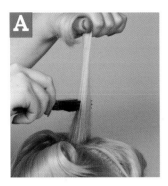

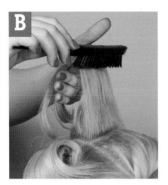

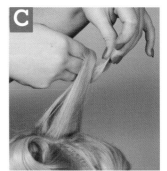

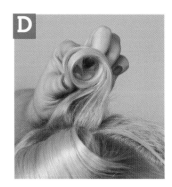

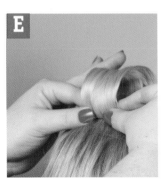

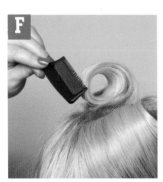

with your fingertips and roll the tube to the scalp, spreading it as you go. (E)

7. Secure the roll with grips.
8. Smooth the roll with a mist of spray, using your fingertips or a brush over the surface to gently remove any stray hairs. (F)

The Faux Victory Roll

The Faux Victory Roll is a simpler version of the Victory Roll, producing a similar silhouette. This style is perfect for when you are finding it hard to attain Victory Rolls, but also for getting another day out of your set while there is still some bend and texture to your hair. The style can be created with or without back-brushing; you simply pull back the hair and slide it forward to add volume. If you do not wish to use back-brushing, simply mist the hair with lots of dry shampoo or back-combing spray.

KIT LIST

Tail comb

Bristle brush

Sectioning clips

Hairpins

Kirby grips

Hairspray

Pomade

Dry shampoo/Back-combing spray

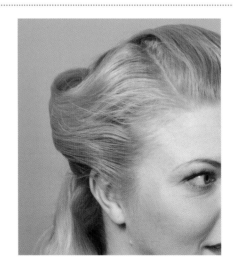

Directions

1. Brush through your hair and section from ear to ear. (A)
2. Spray dry shampoo or back-combing powder throughout the section. (B)
3. Massage through the hair. (C)
4. Take a side section and brush it upwards away from the face. (D)

5. Grip the section firmly between your fingertips and pull it up and away from the face. Press is against the head and then push it forwards and up to meet the parting. This creates volume and the effect of a Victory Roll. (E,F)
6. Make any adjustments to the shape using your fingertips and secure with a comb (you could also use grips). (G)
7. Repeat the process on the opposite side of the head.
8. Smooth the style using your fingertips and a mist of hairspray. Use the end of a tail comb to make any adjustments to the shape.

This style will be easier to recreate on hair that has not been washed for 24–48 hours.

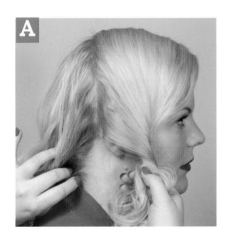

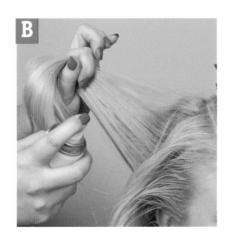

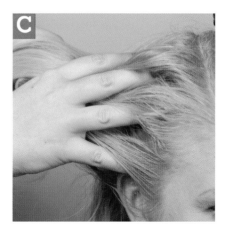

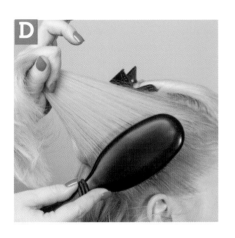

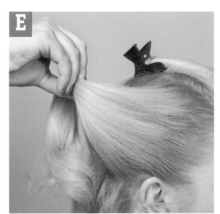

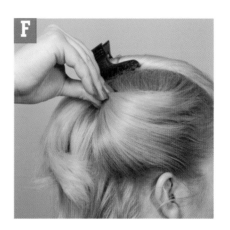

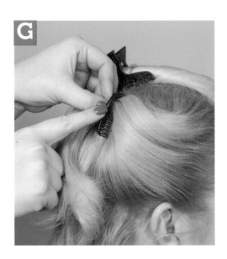

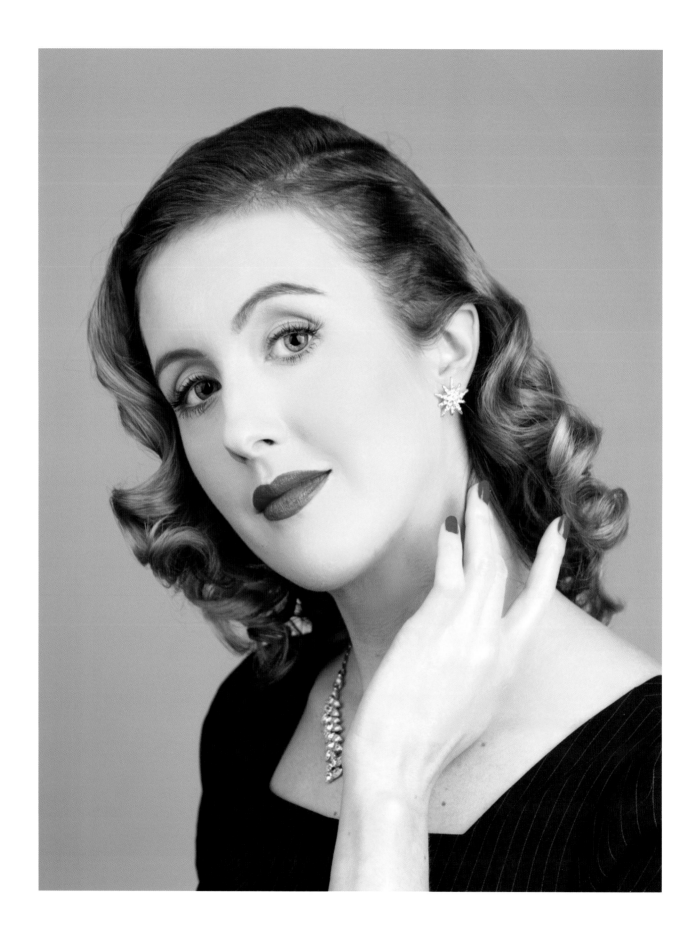

Chapter 5
Brushing Out

5

The Principles of the Brush-out

Regardless of the method you choose, wet or dry, you will need to brush and dress out the set. This is a very important skill and in this chapter I will run through some tips for brushing out different sets and getting the best results.

The most important thing to remember when styling is that your brush is not the only tool used to finish and polish your set; your hands are of great importance too. When brushing out, think of your hands as the principal tool for shaping and moulding the hair. Ultimately, how you work with both your hands and the brush will shape the style.

Think of the silhouette of the style you are trying to achieve; you are moulding the waves and curls into shape, so it helps to have a plan. Have a look at one of your favourite starlets and observe how their waves or curls fall. Are the curls fluffy or smooth? How is the hair shaped around the face? Do the ends flip under or curl out?

Move the brush and your hand in the direction you wish the curls to fall, lie or

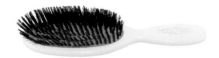

Bristle brush.

bend. Use your fingertips to ping curls into fluff, smooth the hair into glossy waves or shape sections into rolls. No brush can create a fluffy Betty Grable curl or smooth and structure a peek-a-boo wave as well as your hands. Use your fingers to smooth and shape waves

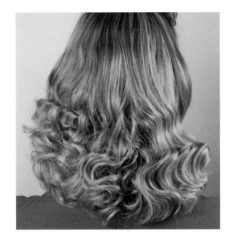

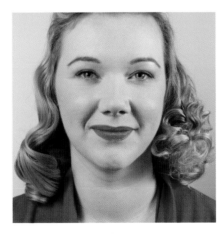

Different curl effects from the same set.

around the face, spreading and holding the dents in waves firmly with one hand as you brush the ends smooth.

Take a look at this finished brush-out. Both of the finishes are from rag curls, rolled in the same direction, but the techniques used to finish the hair have produced two very different effects. The hair on the left of the head was manipulated into textured fluff curls, and on the right, sleek smooth waves. This shows how important the brush-out is in moulding the final result and ultimately how an understanding of the techniques involved will help you achieve the desired result every time.

Pomade helps to work, shape, smooth and hold the hair, so do not forget this step. As you brush out your hair, reapply small amounts to your fingertips as you work.

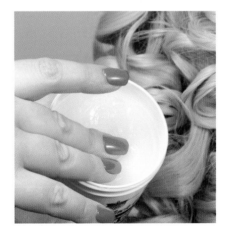

Smooth pomade on your fingertips as you brush out.

Soft-hold hairspray should be used as you brush out, once the very frizzy stage has passed and the style begins to take shape. This will help make the hair more pliable and easier to mould.

I will go over the tips and considerations for brushing out specific sets below. In addition, please see the 'Desired Finishes' section for instructions on how to brush every type of curl set into various finishes, such as waves, fluff curls or sculpted curls.

Brushing out Hot Sets

Compared with the vigorous brush-outs required by wet sets, hot sets do not need as much work.

A combination of natural and synthetic bristles is preferable for most hair types. However, if you have very thick, coarse hair, a nylon styling brush may work better.

Hot Sticks

Hot sticks tend to work well on all hair types. When you take them out they create a tight, fluffy, spiral curl that will need considerable brushing out and can withstand a lot of moulding.

On removal, make sure you unroll the hair from the stick, rather than pulling, to avoid frizz and distorting the curl.

Hot Rollers

Roller sets are best brushed out gently, or if you have very fine hair, using only your fingertips will suffice. Always unroll the rollers gently into coils, as pulling them out may damage the curl.

As roller sets can be a soft curl, first separate the curls with your fingers to minimize the amount of time you have to spend brushing, which can loosen the curl too much. Use a light pomade to avoid weighing down the hair.

Tongs

Tongs produce a good, firm curl on most hair types. The size of tong you use will depend on how much brushing the curls will need.

If you have fine hair, avoid using heavy pomade as this may weigh down the hair too much.

Hot Pin Curls

Hot pin curls have the strongest curl of all the hot sets, so will need more brushing and manipulating.

Ensure you thoroughly break up the sections of hair before you start brushing through and keep your fingers coated with pomade as you work through the hair.

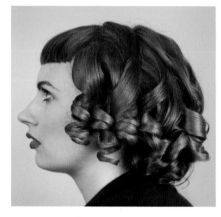

Hot pin curl set.

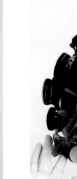

Hot stick curls.

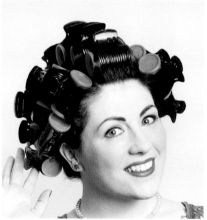

A roller set.

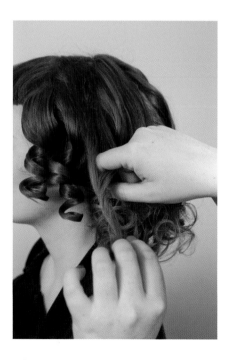

Break up the curls with some pomade.

Brushing out Wet Sets

Wet set curls are very resilient; they can take a lot of moulding and are very malleable. Consequently, they require more brushing and manipulating in order to achieve the desired shape.

When you first try pin curls or another wet set, you will most likely be shocked by the tightness and at times frizziness of the curl as you remove the clips or rollers and begin to brush the hair out. Do not panic. Just keep brushing! Natural bristles can cause lots of frizz when brushing out wet sets, so I recommend a nylon styling brush with strong, firm teeth for lots of control.

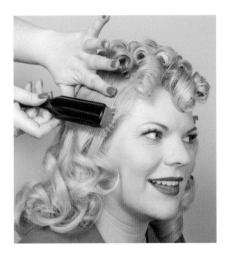

Brushing out a wet set.

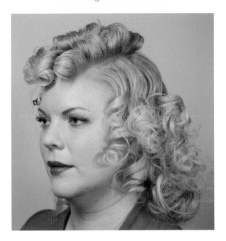

Wet set frizz.

The amount of time spent brushing through a pin curl or wet set until it reaches the desired effect is much longer than needed for a hot set as the curl is more dense.

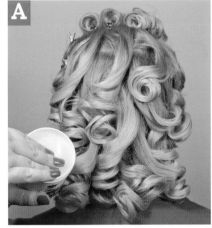

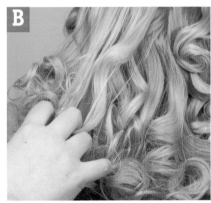

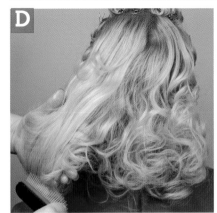

Directions

1. Start by removing all the rollers, rags or pin curl clips. Initially, the curls will be very springy, in ringlets, and the hair will appear considerably shorter as a result.

2. Before you start brushing, separate the curls with your fingers and begin to break them up. A small slick of pomade on your fingers helps this process and prepares the hair for the brush-out by adding hold and control, and smoothing the hair. (A,B,C)

3. Once the hair is a bit looser and broken up, you can begin to brush through the set.

4. At this point, the hair will be very dense and will become frizzy and

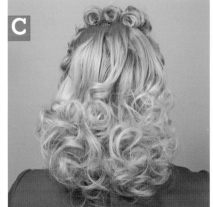

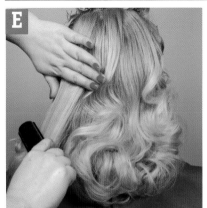

big. Don't be alarmed: the only solution is to keep on brushing. Instead of just brushing the hair with the brush alone, brush the hair together with and onto your hand to control the frizz. (D)

5. Another technique for smoothing the hair and combatting frizz is to smooth your hand down the section of hair as you brush. (E)

After an initial brush-through, start brushing the hair in the direction you wish it to sit. For example, if you would like the curls in a big smooth wave towards the face, think about this shape as you brush, train the hair in this direction, smooth it onto your hand and towards the face. If you want all of the hair to be tucked under into a sleek pageboy, concentrate on smoothing the crown with your hand and brushing the hair underneath. If you are trying to create fluff curls, brush through the hair but then separate into fluff curls with your fingers. If you are trying to create waves, work on moulding the hair together into one piece.

See the specific sections on brushing into waves, fluff and sculptured curls for guidance on achieving your specific, desired finish.

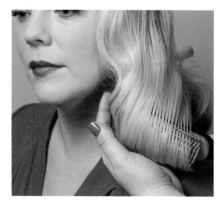

Smoothing the hair.

TIP

- Using a spritz of soft-hold hairspray while dressing out helps shape the waves by making the hair more pliable.
- Use clips to shape the waves.
- Don't forget – your fingers are a useful shaping tool.
- If your hair is still very frizzy, smooth any flyaway hairs by finishing with another application of light serum or pomade, ensuring you work it right to the ends of the hair.
- Experiment with different brushes to find the best for your hair type.

How to Brush into your Desired Finish

Waves

Directions

1. Separate through the curls using your fingertips and some pomade. (A)
2. Firmly brush the curls together, repeatedly brushing each section down onto your hand, moulding the hair into one and smoothing the ends together. A mist of soft-hold hairspray will make the hair more pliable and help you work it into the desired shape. (B)
3. You will start to see the natural wave appear as you release tension from the hair and let it fall naturally. Keep brushing and moulding the hair together. (C,D)
4. Pay attention to the crown too, smoothing any gaps. (E)
5. Use curl clips to accentuate any waves. (F)
6. Move onto the sides of the head, brushing the hair firmly down onto your hand, joining it together into one section of hair. Ensure you pay attention to the ends of the hair,

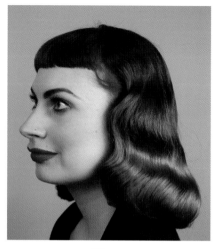

Waves.

smoothing them together and removing frizz. (G)

7. Brush them down into one section, and with the hair taut, grasp the hair firmly between the fingertips. Still holding the hair firmly, release the tension. You will see the hair start to spring into its natural wave. (H,I,J)
8. Let the hair lie in this shape, spreading the bottom of the wave gently outwards. (K)
9. Gently join the front section to the back, brushing it together and closing any gaps. (L)
10. Use your fingers to firmly hold the hair in the wave indent whilst you work on smoothing out the waves below. (M,N)
11. You can also use duck-billed clips to hold the hair in place as you work. (O)
12. Once you are happy with the shape, place a small amount of pomade on your hands and smooth over the style with your palms and fingertips. Long metal pin curl/duck-billed clips can be used to accentuate the wave by clipping the wave dents and misting with spray. Leave the spray to dry and remove the clips. (P,Q)

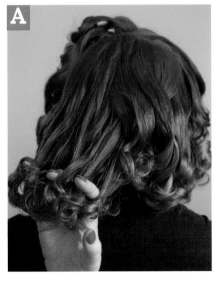

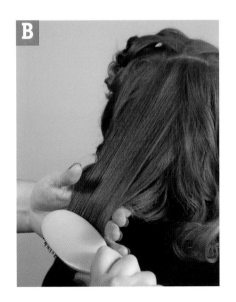

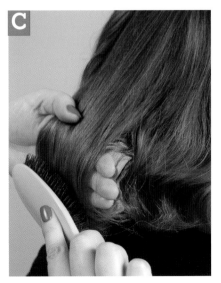

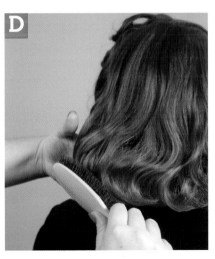

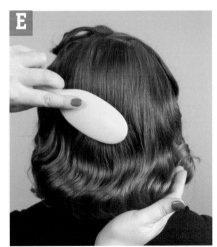

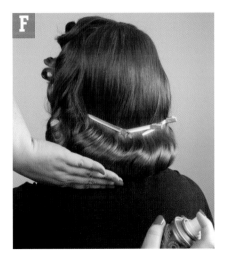

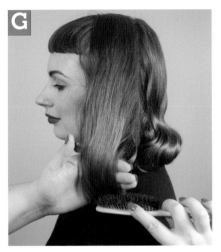

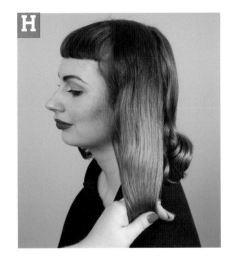

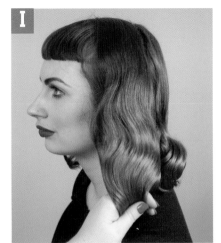

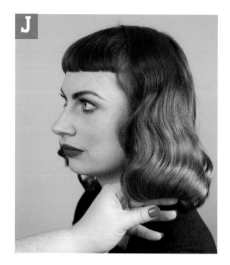

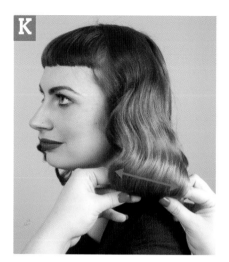

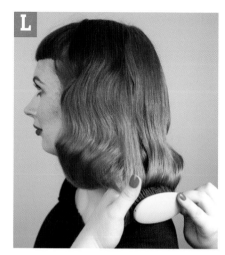

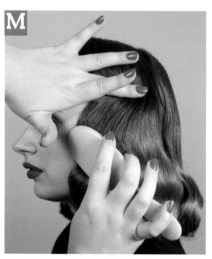

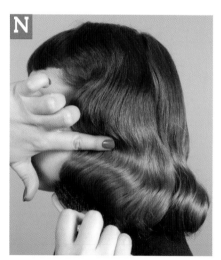

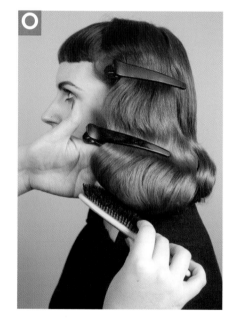

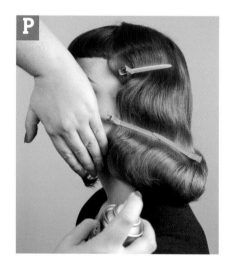

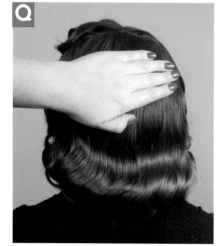

Unified Wave Technique

This method helps to pull curls together and brush them into a smooth wave. It works very well on moulding the back section of hair into a uniformed wave, but also works on the side sections.

Directions

1. Coat you fingers with some pomade. Pull the hair back as if you were styling it into a ponytail, brushing the hair into one piece. (A)
2. Make sure you also brush the ends together. (B)
3. Loosen your grip on the hair slightly and pull the hand holding your hair downwards slowly, right to the bottom, letting the hair drop naturally from your hand. (C,D,E)
4. Use your fingertips to gently spread the wave. (F)
5. If the hair has a lot of breaks, repeat the process until you are satisfied with the effect. A mist of soft-hold hairspray while you work will help make the hair more pliable.
6. Use your hands to smooth and shape the hair. (G)

This is a soft wave, as we used large pin curls.

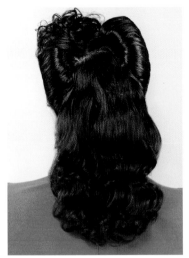

This is the result of the same technique on 1cm thick hot sticks.

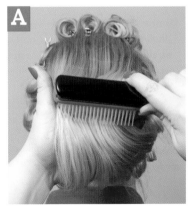

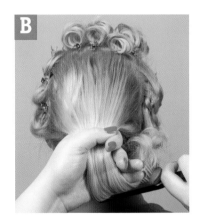

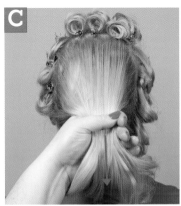

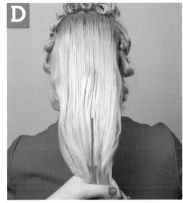

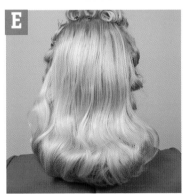

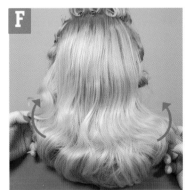

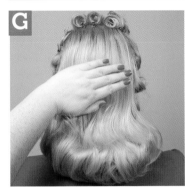

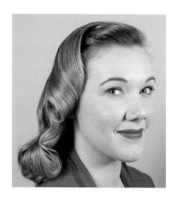
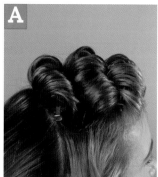
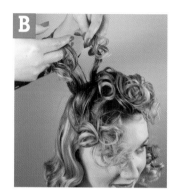
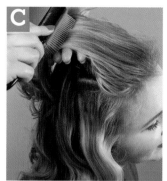

S-Wave

This sleek front detail works with many styles and lengths.

Directions

1. To set, roll all the hair in the crown section away from the face on base. Here we used stand-up pin curls, but any curling technique could be used. (A)
2. Once set, separate the curls. If you have fine hair, you could add some back-brushing to the roots at this point. (B)
3. Smooth the section away from the face. (C)
4. Pay attention to the ends, brushing them back towards the face, while maintaining the natural curve the hair will fall into, the first curve of the S. A mist of soft-hold hairspray while you work will help make the hair more pliable. (D)
5. Use a finger to hold the top section, sweeping backwards as you smooth the lower section forwards to accentuate the S shape. (E)
6. Use hairspray to help you shape the hair. (F)
7. Use your fingers and clips to accentuate the S shape and make any adjustments. (G)
8. Mist with hairspray and secure with pins.

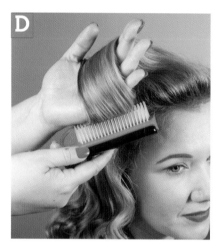
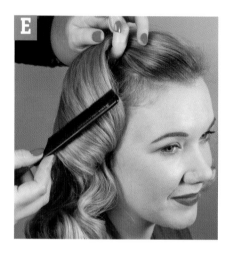
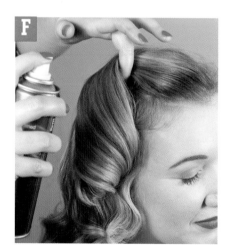
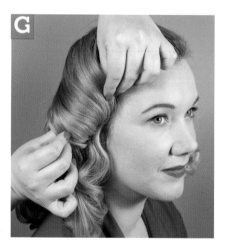

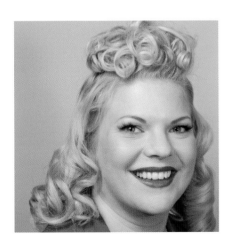

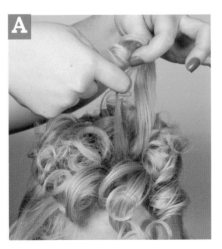

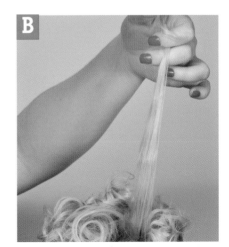

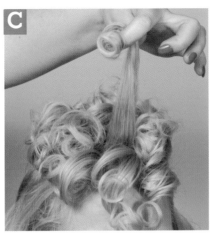

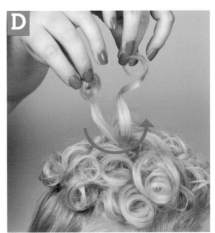

Defined Fluff Curls

Fluff curls are best created with a tighter curl. For a defined look, fluff can be created directly from a curl without brushing.

Directions

1. With pomade on your fingertips, separate each curl into smaller curls, pulling each one upwards, applying tension and then releasing, letting it ping into shape. (A,B,C)
2. Add structure to the curls by knitting them together. (D)
3. Using hairpins rather than grips will help maintain the soft, loose nature of the fluff as they will not squash the curls as much. If more securing is required, use bent hairpins.

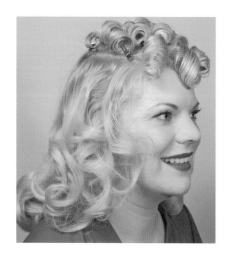

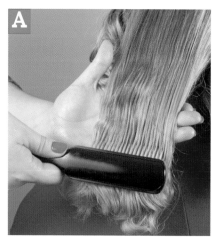

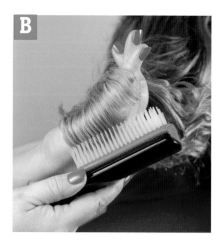

Soft Fluff Curls

Directions

1. Separate the curls using your fingertips and some pomade. If you are brushing out a hot set, this may be all you need to produce a soft fluff curl. If your hair is set in a wet set or you have naturally curly or frizzy hair, then continue to the next step.
2. Brush the curls together onto your hand, making sure you brush through the ends thoroughly. (A,B)
3. You should see the hair become smoother and the frizz disappear from the ends of the hair. (C)
4. Next, comb through the hair with your fingertips, separating the hair into fluff curls. (D,E)

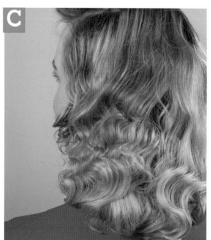

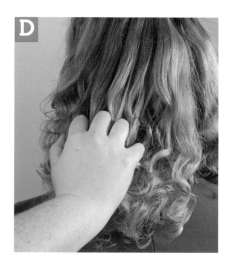

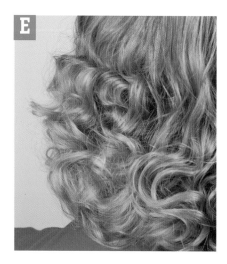

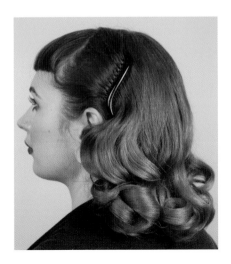

Sculpted Curls

Directions

1. Separate the curls using your fingertips and some pomade.

2. Start brushing through the curls. (A) Concentrate on smoothing the hair, brushing the hair onto your hand and removing any frizz. A mist of soft-hold hairspray while you work will help make the hair more pliable. (B)

3. Add more pomade to your fingertips and start dividing the hair into sections. Brush each section around your fingertip to smooth and ensure the ends are free from frizz. (C,D)

4. Pull each section away from the head and let the hair slide off and fall into its natural shape. Repeat for each section until you achieve the desired finish. (E,F,G)

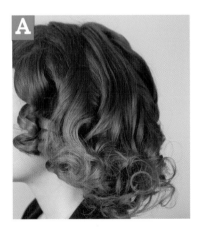

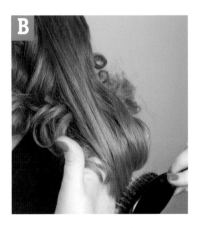

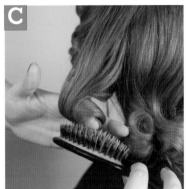

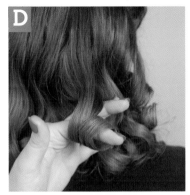

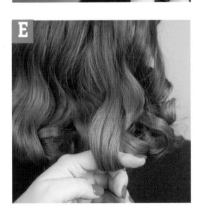

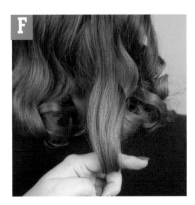

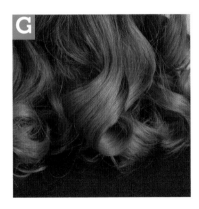

Finger Waves

Directions

1. Brush through the hair, ensuring the brush makes good contact with the scalp. If the bristles are facing away from the head, it will pull the hair away, creating loose, frizzy curls. Brushing with all the bristles facing the same way and connecting fully with the scalp creates a smoother, neater wave. Use your fingertips to hold the ridges as you brush out the wave below. (A)

2. Push the waves upwards with the side of your hand to accentuate any ridges. (B,C)

3. Accentuate ridges with clips and hairspray. (D)

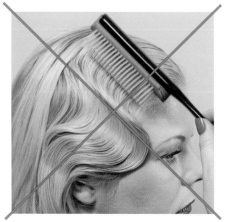

Make sure the bristles stay in contact with your head as you brush.

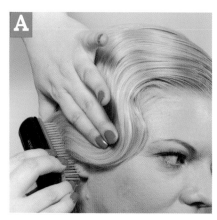

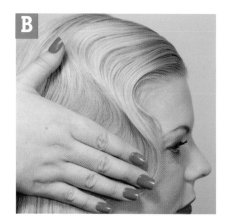

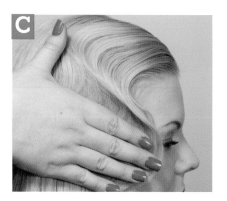

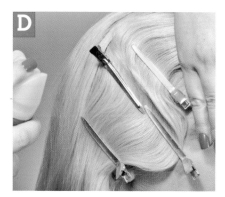

Extra Tips and Tricks

Crossed Grips

Crossed grips are used to create a firm foundation within a hairstyle. They are used in styles such as the Gibson Roll to hold the hair securely as Barrel Rolls are formed.

The technique of criss-crossing locks the pins in place and stops them moving around or lifting the hair below.

Directions

1. Brush through the section to be pinned and smooth it down with a mist of hairspray. (A)
2. Hold the hair flat with one hand and secure the hair with a grip, ensuring you catch the lower layers. Interlock the next pin, making sure it crosses the first. (B,C)
3. Continue pinning in this way, holding the hair flat. (D)

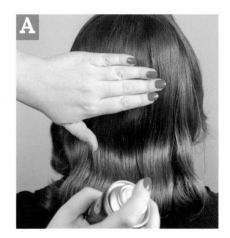

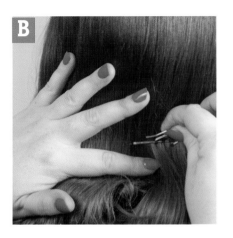

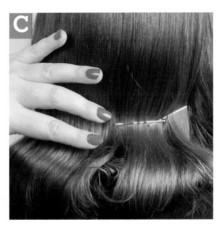

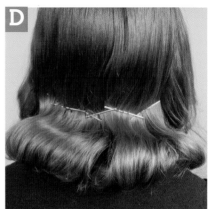

Blending With Hairpins

Hairpins are used to bridge and close any splits in the hair contained in rolls, pompadours and other parts of your style.

Directions

1. Use the prongs of a hairpin to close the gap. (A,B)
2. Mist with hairspray. (C)
3. Allow to dry for as long as possible and remove the pins.

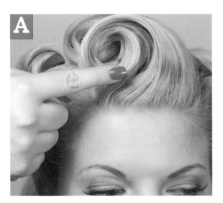

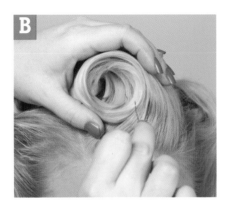

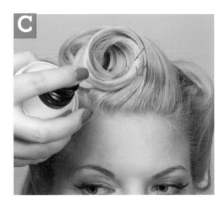

Shaping With Clips

Pin curl and duck-billed clips are perfect for helping you mould your finished style. Use them to make adjustments to the shape and hold sections of the hair in place as you work through others.

Misting clipped sections with a light mist of hairspray, leaving to dry and then removing the clips helps hold the style in place and also accentuates specific waves and curls within the style.

Ridged duck-billed clips are perfect for controlling thick hair.

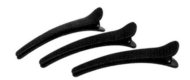

Ridged duck billed clip.

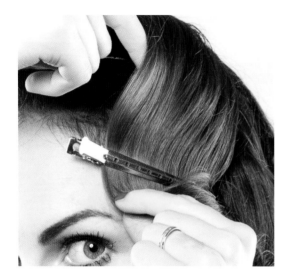
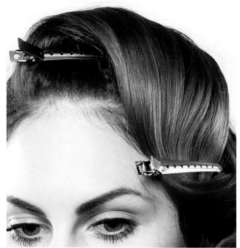
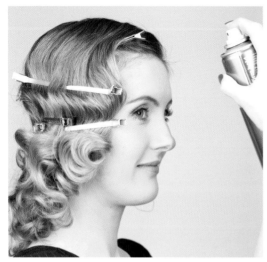
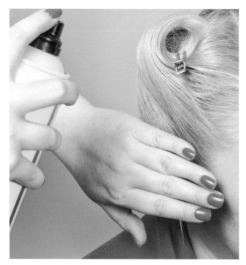

Different ways of using clips to shape your style.

How to Refresh your Set

Regardless of your hair type, there will come a time when your curls start to drop. For some lucky ladies, a pin curl set can last a few days until you wash the curls out. For others, the bounce and curl may last only one or two days at most.

If you wish to prolong your set, you can pin it back up dry rather than repeating the whole process. Roll the hair back up into flat pin curls or around sponge rollers. Keep it dry or lightly mist the set with water (no setting lotion should be used this time as it will overload the hair with product). Sleep on the pinned set and brush out the next morning. The set will need much less thorough brushing than the original pin curl set.

If the curls are down and they seem a bit frizzy, brush through the set again with pomade to refresh the style.

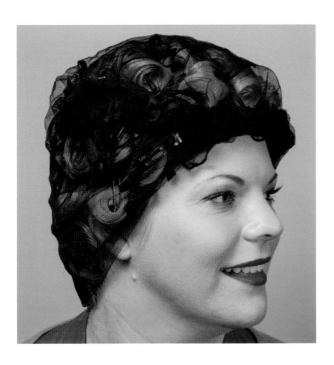

4 TOP TIPS FOR A LASTING SET

1. Don't get it wet.
2. Re-roll it at night.
3. Wear a slumber net or headscarf to bed.
4. Wear a shower cap in the shower or bath to avoid your hair being exposed to steam/splashes of water.

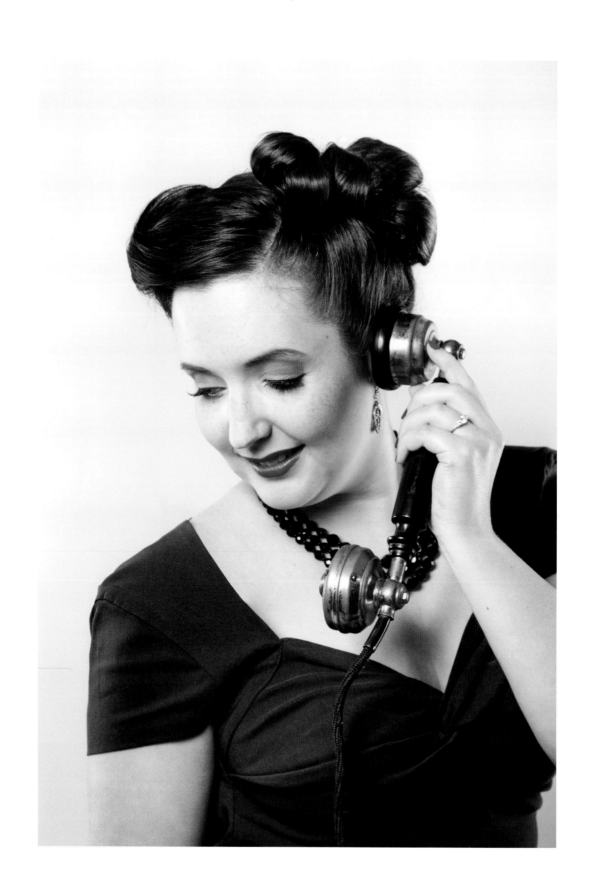

Chapter 6
Step-by-step Guide to Classic Up Styles

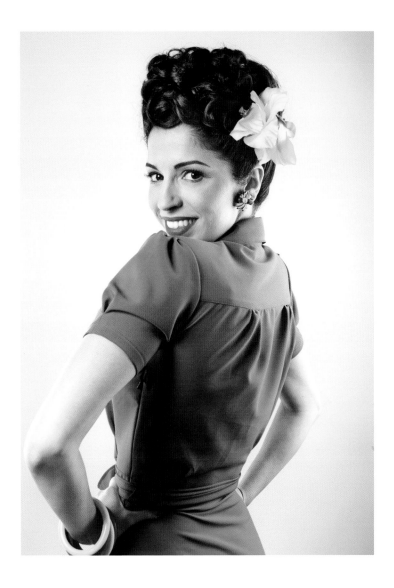

The next two chapters provide instructions for more than 30 authentic 1940s hairstyles, inspired by the glamorous starlets and the most popular trends of the period. These styles and their instructions are designed to be used in conjunction with the 'Creating Curls' and 'Brushing Out' chapters. Each specific method you will need to create every style is listed along with a tutorial, so please take a moment to familiarize yourself with the techniques required for each style before proceeding.

Modern methods are used for many of these looks, but remember: every style that involves creating curl comes with its own pin curl pattern if you wish to use a traditional wet set (see Appendix). Therefore, select the technique that suits you. The looks can be adapted to your own hair length, texture and personal taste, so be sure to experiment and create the style that's perfect for you.

The Pin-Up

Also known as The Poodle, this style was popularized by Betty Grable and also Lucille Ball.

The hair at the side of the hair was pulled up flat, whilst the hair on the crown lay in a mass of curls. This style was worn in many ways, from smooth, sculpted curls to textured and fluffy curls. This look is based upon Betty's iconic bathing suit pose from 1942, which portrays the star glancing coquettishly over her shoulder. Reportedly, around 5 million copies of this image were distributed to soldiers overseas to keep up morale.

As Betty's famous style had a lot of height, I used an extra-large hair rat, but you can use a smaller size or work with your own hair to produce a more toned-down look. This style looks stunning dressed up with a sparkly clip or brooch pinned to the front for evening elegance, or a flower would work for daytime.

Directions

1. Divide the hair into four sections. (A,B)
2. Pin the three lower sections flat onto the head. Smooth with a brush as you go and try to avoid any gaps. Spraying the sections with hairspray helps control the hair. Fix each section with crossed pins, holding the hair down firmly with one hand and securing with the other, making sure you pick up the lower layers of hair as well as the top section as you slide in the pins. The hair is divided into three sections for ease, but you could do all three at once if you prefer. (C,D,E)
3. Once the hair is pinned, roll the hair around the hot sticks randomly in different directions, following no fixed pattern. Remember not to put too much hair on each hot stick, as you want to achieve a very strong, bouncy curl. (F)
4. Once they have cooled completely, remove the hot sticks. (G)
5. Part the curls and grip a doughnut or some stuffing in the centre. (H)
6. Divide each section into multiple fluff curls and pin the curls randomly to the crown and hair sponge, knitting them together loosely to make them secure. (I,J)

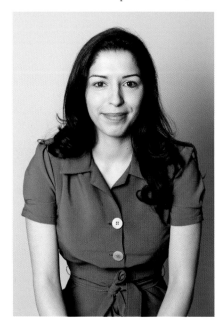

Shown on model with long hair.

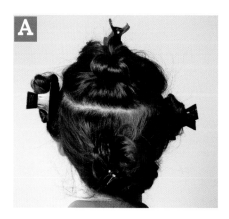

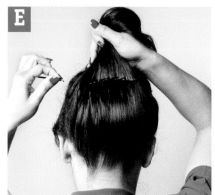

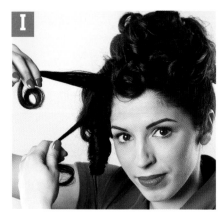

7. Make sure you cover all of the padding and use the curls to cover the Kirby grips at the back and sides of the head. Hairpins are useful at this point as they blend more easily into the hair and do not flatten the curl as much as Kirby grips. (K)
8. Finish the style with a mist of hairspray.

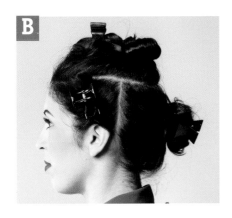

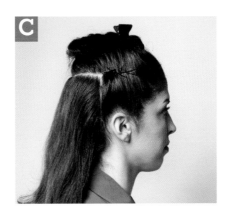

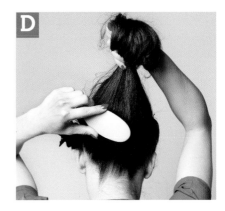

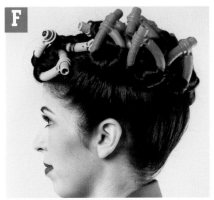

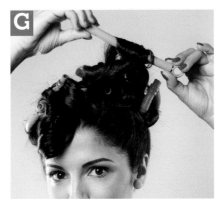

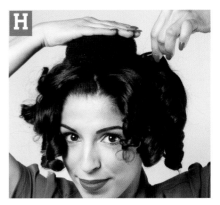

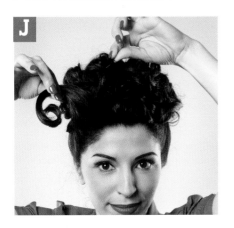

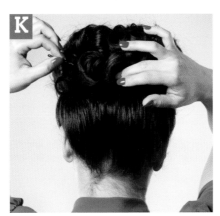

The French Bun

This sleek and sophisticated up style is simple to achieve. It can be created if the hair is sufficiently long to be pulled into a high ponytail, as clip-in extensions can be added beneath the bun if more length is required.

Although it is perfect for evening glamour, it looks equally stunning with a day dress.

TECHNIQUES REQUIRED

Hot rollers

KIT LIST

Bristle brush
Hair elastic
Kirby grips
Hairpins
Pomade
Hairspray
Hot rollers (1–1.25 inch)

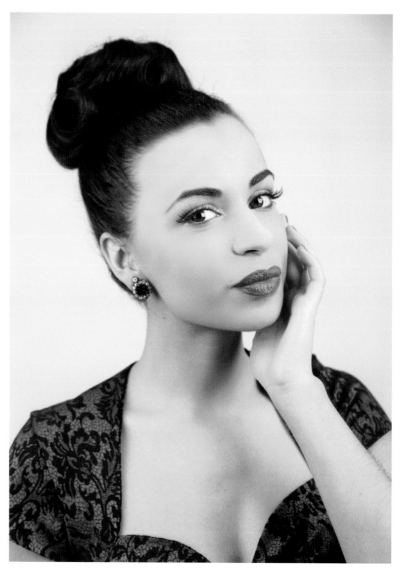

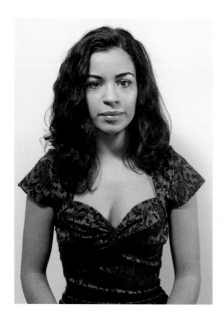

Shown on model with medium-length hair.

Directions

1. Brush the hair into a high ponytail. (A)
2. Smooth any flyaway hairs. (B)
3. Set the hair in hot rollers, leaving to cool completely. (C,D)
4. Remove the rollers. (E)
5. Add a synthetic doughnut over the ponytail. (F)
6. Form the hair into pin curls, spreading them to cover the stuffing. (G,H,I,J)
7. Pin into place. (K)
8. Continue working around until the doughnut is completely covered. There is no pattern to this; the curls are pinned randomly. (L)
9. Apply a mist of hairspray and use a tail comb to smooth any flyaway hairs. (M)

TIP

Alternative curling methods: A large-barrelled tong could create the curls. If you wish to use a wet set, Velcro or foam rollers may be used.

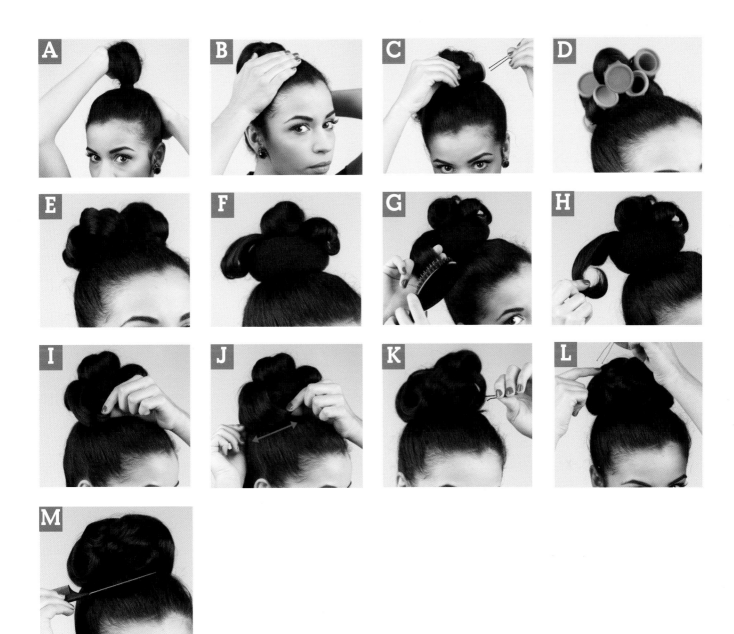

The Carmen

Inspired by screen legend Carmen Miranda, this fun, daytime style is perfect for giving short hair a 1940s look in no time at all, although it can work on all lengths of hair.

If you have no fringe, you can still set the curls in the same way; after curling, simply roll the hair into a series of sculpted curls and secure with grips. On long hair, this method is perfect for transitioning the style from day to night, as the elevated pin curls can be brushed into a nice wave for the evening. For this alternative look, prepare the hair underneath the scarf at the back with pin curls and leave to set.

TECHNIQUES USED

Sculpted curls

Shaping with clips

How to tie a headscarf

KIT LIST

Hot sticks (0.5 in/13mm)

Pomade

Sectioning clips

Hairspray

Curl clips

Kirby grips

Tail comb/Bristle brush

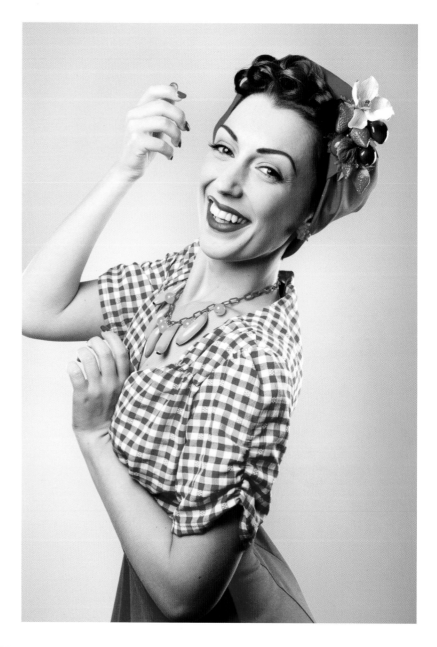

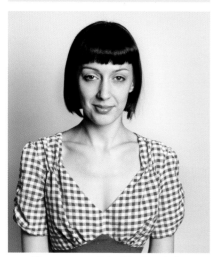

Shown on model with short hair.

Directions

1. Set the fringe/front section of your hair in hot sticks, using end papers to help control the ends of the hair. Leave the hot sticks to cool completely. (A,B,C)
2. Remove and separate the curls into elevated pin curls. (D,E)
3. Use pin curl clips to help form the curls. This is achieved by using the clips to hold the curl in the desired shape and spraying with a strong-hold hairspray to set the curl. Wait for the spray to dry and remove the clips. Mist with another fine layer of spray. (F)
4. Add a headscarf or turban to finish the look. (See Chapter 8 for tutorials.)

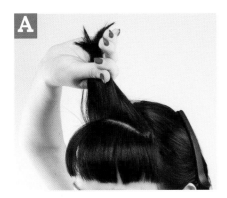

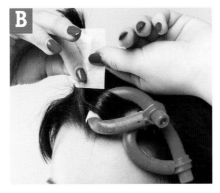

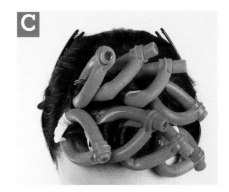

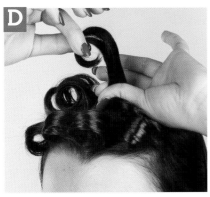

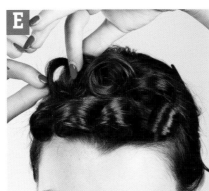

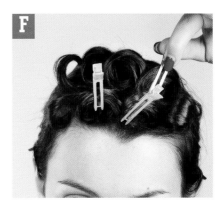

The Rosie

This style, inspired by the legendary 'Rosie the Riveter', is a quick style that can be achieved in minimum time and without pre-curling. The look is finished with a headscarf, but you could wear the back in a variety of ways, up or down. It is the perfect style for wearing out and about with a drying pin curl set wrapped up in the scarf.

TECHNIQUES REQUIRED

Use of a rat/padding

KIT LIST

Hairgrips
Foam doughnut/rat
Bristle brush
Pomade
Hairspray

You can purchase foam doughnuts that can be opened out with buttons on the ends; these are perfect as they already have rounded edges. Alternatively you can cut a doughnut in half, but you must gather and sew the ends together to create a round edge (this is because a square edge is tricky to blend into the hair).

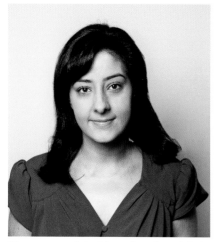

Shown on model with medium-length hair.

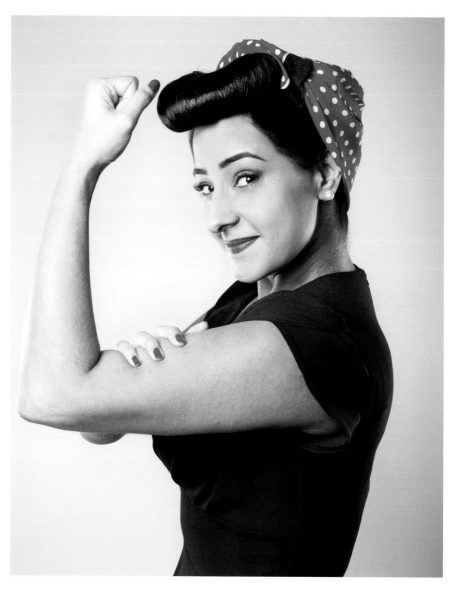

Directions

1. Section off a circular section of hair at the front of the head. This is taken from above the arch of each brow and to the top of the crown. (A)
2. Pull the hair horizontally from the head and place the sponge a few centimetres from the forehead. Wrap the hair around the sponge, keeping the hair taut. (B,C)
3. Tuck in the ends and twist under the hair and sponge to tighten. (D)
4. Roll the sponge towards the face until it sits at the desired height. Experiment and see what height looks best for you. (E)
5. Pull up the ends of the sponge and place against the scalp so that they sit just above the partings in the hair. (F)
6. Keeping a firm hold at all times, fix the sponge in place with grips until it feels secure. (G)
7. Gently spread the hair over the sponge with your fingertips. (H,I)
8. A tail comb can also help to distribute the hair and tuck and

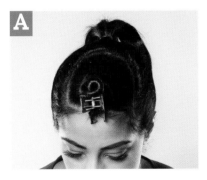

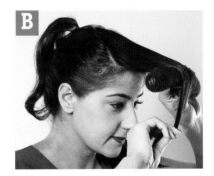

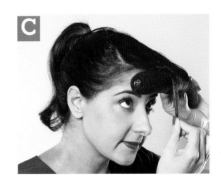

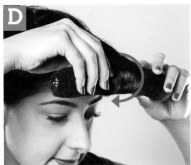

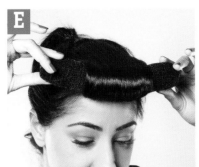

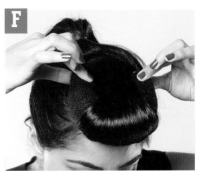

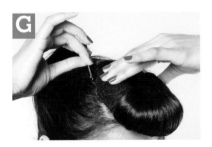

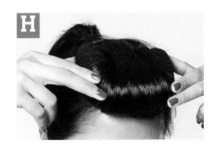

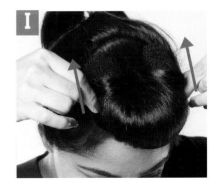

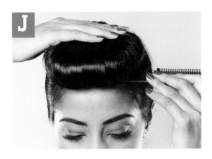

loose strands underneath the roll. (J)

9. Pin into place.

10. Finish with a mist of hairspray, using the tail comb to tuck any loose strands under the roll whilst the hair is still tacky.

11. Add a headscarf or snood to complete the look.

TIP

I have a fringe: This style can still work for you. Pull some long pieces of hair forward from the back of your head and roll them with the fringe. If you find that your fringe keeps dropping out as you try to roll your hair around the sponge, simply add some teasing and hairspray. This will make it easier to tuck in the fringe. Do not tease the whole section – just the fringe – as if you do, it will make it hard to spread the hair smoothly over the roll.

My fringe roll is floppy: You have to maintain good tension on the fringe as you roll it. If at any point it feels loose, simply twist the roll under to tighten the hair around it before you continue rolling to the forehead.

The Braided Coronet

Worn by the starlet Dorothy Lamour, the rope braid is a classic 1940s style that is easy to reproduce. This regal style is created from a braided hairpiece, but if your hair is long and thick, you could create it from your own hair.

The hairpiece is simple to make, and by making it yourself you have the benefit of matching it perfectly to your hair colour.

TECHNIQUES USED

How to make a braided hairpiece:
rope braiding

KIT LIST

Braided hairpiece
Clear hair elastic
Hairgrips
Hairpins
Bristle brush
Gel (optional)

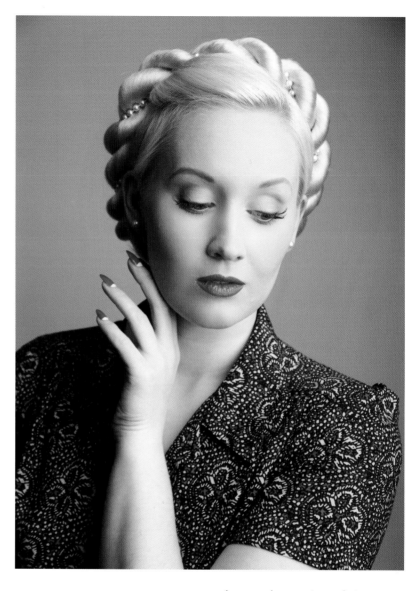

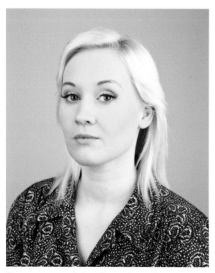

Shown on model with medium-length hair.

Directions

1. Follow the instructions for creating a rope braid as detailed in the 'Completing the Look' chapter. Make a braided hairpiece that matches your hair colour and measure it against your head to get the correct length. Alternatively see the tips box for creating the braid from your own hair.

2. With your hair in a side parting, add a small amount of back-brushing to the centre-front section and pin to achieve a small amount of lift and volume. Alternatively, you could have the hair brushed back, completely sleek. (A,B)

3. Smooth your hair into a low ponytail and mist with hairspray, smoothing any flyaway hairs. (C)

4. Grip one end of the hairpiece securely so it sits directly on top of the ponytail. (D)

5. Wrap the other end of the hairpiece around the head, at the back on top

of the ponytail so the braid forms a
complete circle. (E)

6. Divide the ends of the ponytail in
   two and tuck and grip the ends
   under the braid. If your hair is very
   thick, twisting the hair firmly will
   make the section smaller and easier
   to pin. (F)

7. Use hairpins in an anchoring motion
   to secure the braid around the head.
   (G)

TIP

My braid is fluffy: Smooth any stray
hairs on the braid with a small amount of
gel.

Instructions for using your own hair: If
your hair is very long (to the middle of
your back or longer), you can start the
braid in a ponytail at the top of your
head. If your hair is shorter then create
two pigtail bunches and create a rope
braid on each one, securing them
together at the crown. Follow the
instructions for creating a rope braid in
the 'Completing the Look' chapter.

To create a smooth braid: Have a small
amount of gel on your hands as you
braid. This will give you a smooth plait.

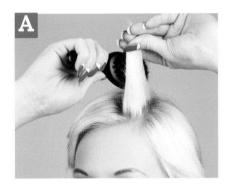

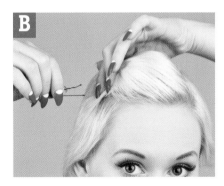

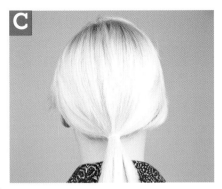

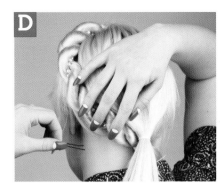

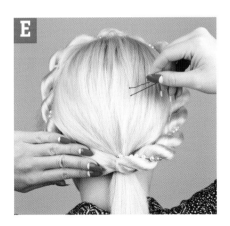

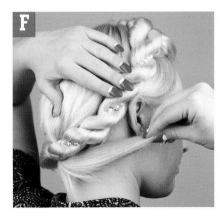

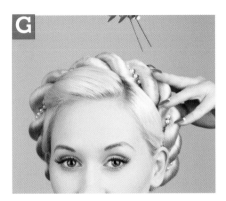

Braided Chignon

This beautiful style also uses a braided hairpiece and demonstrates how a chignon can be created quickly and easily. Any type of braid can be used and it will work on any length of hair, as long as it can be pulled back into a ponytail.

If you have very long, thick hair, a chignon can be created using your own hair. Simply braid and wrap the hair around the base of the braid to form the chignon. The tutorial to create this hairpiece can be found in the 'Completing the Look' chapter.

Directions

1. Tie the hair into a ponytail according to the height at which you wish the chignon to sit. On the last wrap of the band, do not pull all the

---

TECHNIQUES USED

How to make a braided hairpiece:
rope braid

Kit List
Braided hairpiece
Kirby grips
Hairpins
Hairspray
Gel (optional)

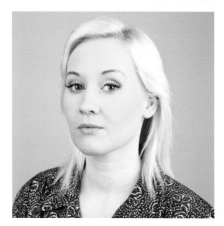

Shown on model with medium-length hair.

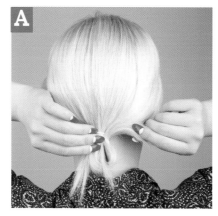

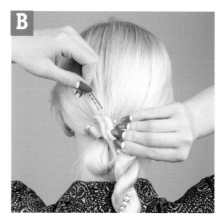

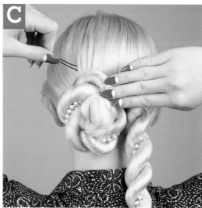

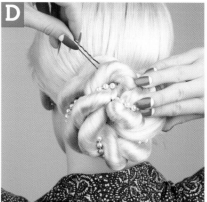

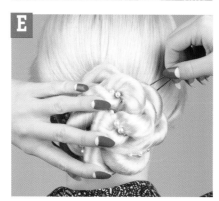

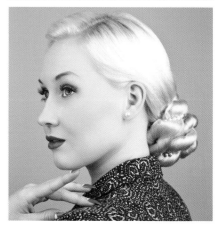

The finished look.

hair quite through, leaving you with a loop. (A)
2. Take the end of the braided hairpiece and grip it securely to the head. (B)
3. Wrap the hair around the ponytail, gripping it as you go. (C)

4. Continue this process until you reach the end, and then grip it over the middle of the chignon. (D)
5. Use hairpins and grips to anchor and secure the chignon in place. (E)
6. Smooth the flat section of hair using your hand and some hairspray.

Topped with a Bow

This pretty bow can be dressed up for evening elegance or accessorized with flowers and paired with a summer dress. Simple to achieve, it requires no pre-curling and can be created in a matter of minutes.

TECHNIQUES REQUIRED

Barrel Rolls

KIT LIST

Bristle brush
Hair elastic
Hairpins
Kirby grips
Hairspray
Pomade

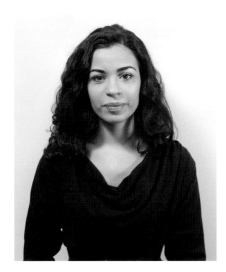

Shown on model with medium-length hair.

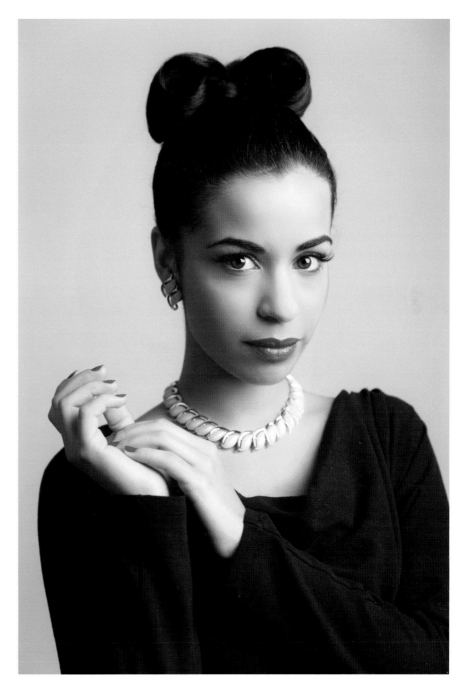

Directions

1. Brush the hair into a high ponytail. (A)
2. Take a small section of hair and wrap it around the base of the ponytail, covering the elastic and securing with a pin. (B,C,D)
3. Mist the section with hairspray and smooth with your fingertips. (E)
4. Split the hair into two and clip one side out of the way. (F)
5. Add back-brushing throughout the first section. (G)
6. Smooth the top layer and roll around your fingers into a Barrel Roll. (H,I)
7. Once it is resting on the head, spread the roll with your fingertips. (J)
8. Pin into place, and then repeat the process on the opposite side. (K)

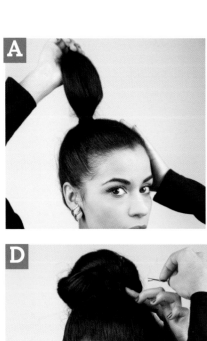

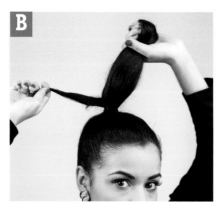

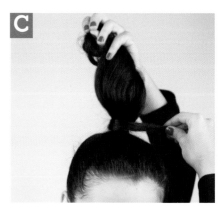

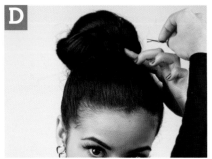

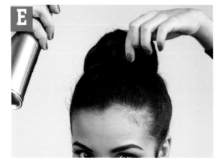

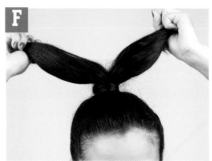

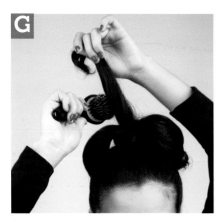

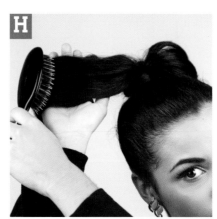

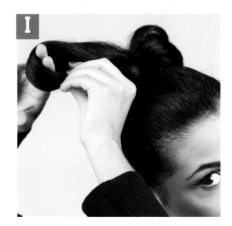

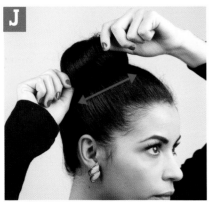

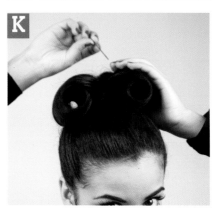

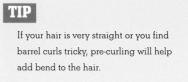

TIP

If your hair is very straight or you find barrel curls tricky, pre-curling will help add bend to the hair.

Make Do and Mend

This style shows how authentic looks can be created quickly and without always having to curl the hair. It is perfect for creating a great look in minimum time.

For this style, you need to create your own snood. Lace with a small amount of stretch was used as it is easy to pin into and a bit of stretch allows it to be manipulated into the desired shape. Alternatively, dress the back of the hair with curls.

The model illustrating this style has a fringe, but it would work without one and on any length of hair, providing there is sufficient length to roll into a pin curl.

TECHNIQUES REQUIRED

Pin curls (dry)
Faux Victory Roll

KIT LIST

Kit List
Lace/fabric
Kirby grips
Hairpins
Hairspray
Pomade

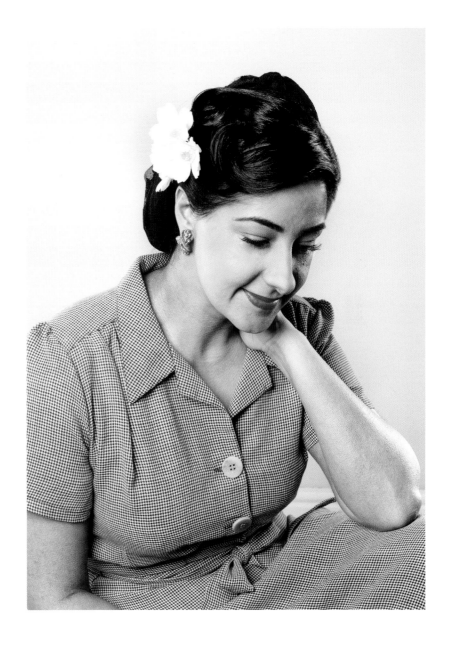

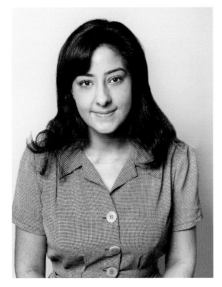

Shown on model with medium-length hair.

Directions

1. Make a parting from ear to ear. Divide the section in front of the ears into four whilst forming one large section at the back. (A,B)
2. Create Faux Victory Rolls with the side sections, securing both with a comb or pin. (C,D)
3. Back-brush one of the crown sections, then smooth and form into a large pin curl. Roll it around your fingers and to the head as you would a wet pin curl and grip in to place. (E,F)
4. Repeat this process with the remaining crown section, securing both sections with grips. (G)
5. Mist the style with hairspray.

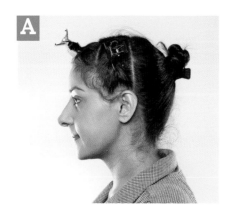

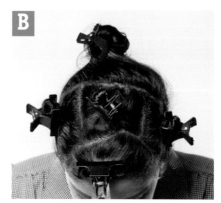

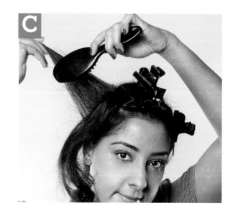

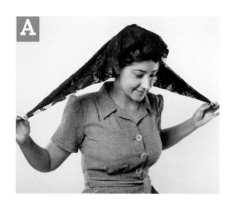

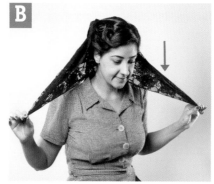

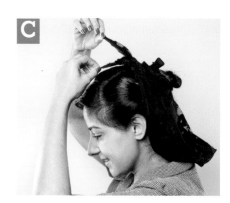

Creating a Snood from Fabric

1. Keeping the back in a sectioning clip, take your large scarf or piece of fabric. Fold the fabric or scarf to make a large triangle.
2. Lay it on the head so the point of the triangle sits over the forehead. (A)
3. Gently pull the fabric down the head so the straight section rests on the back of the neck. (B)
4. Tie the two ends in a knot at the crown of the head. The folded fabric will create a natural pocket at the nape of the neck. (C)

5. Open this out with your hands and unclip your hair, guiding it into the pocket in the fabric. (D,E)
6. Roll and tuck the fabric and hair inwards together. (F,G,H,I)
7. Once you are happy with the roll, secure with hairpins, using an anchoring motion. (J)

This style could be created with a knitted snood or headscarf, keeping the front section styled in the same way.

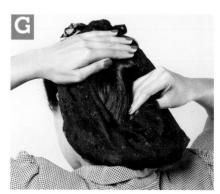

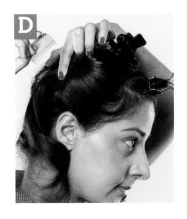

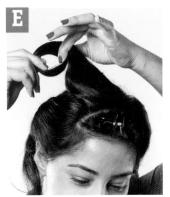

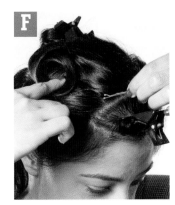

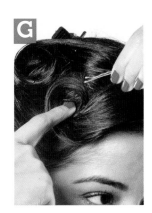

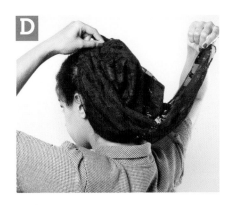

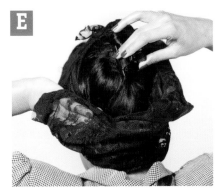

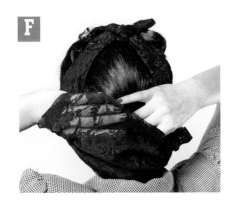

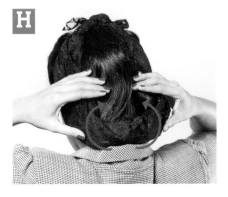

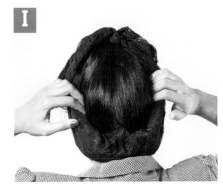

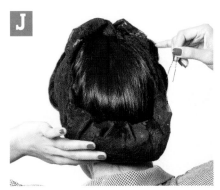

Braided Elegance

This elegant style works well for both day and night. It is stunning when accessorized with flowers or studded with pearls or jewels for the evening. Twists at the sides sweep down the head into a woven roll at the back. This style uses no heat and is quick and easy to recreate.

TECHNIQUES REQUIRED

Plaiting

KIT LIST

Hairgrips
Pomade
Hairspray
Hair bands
Detangling brush/styling brush

Directions

1. Locate where you would like your parting and let the hair fall naturally. Give it a good brush through to remove any tangles.
2. Take a small section of hair from the front of the head and twist it away from the face. (A)

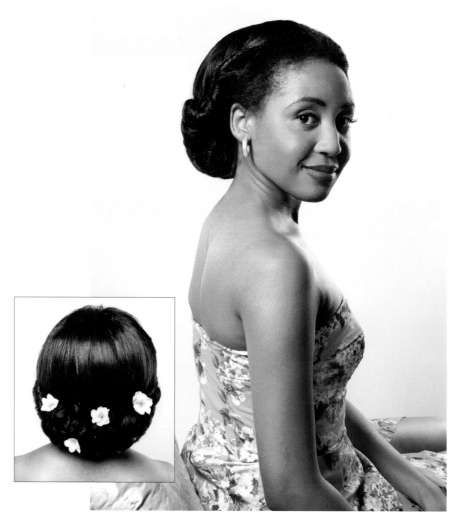

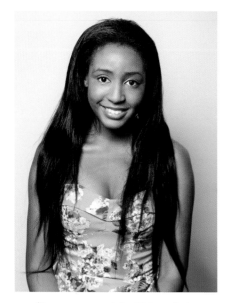

Shown on a model with long hair.

3. Take another section of hair from just underneath the previous section and twist these together away from the face in the same direction. (B,C)
4. Repeat this until you get a larger section of hair, picking up sections of hair as you go and taking care not to let go and let the strands untwist. (D,E)
5. Keep going until you reach the back of the head, securing the centre of the roll with grips and pins until it feels secure. (F,G)
6. Repeat the process on the other side of the head. (H)

7. Divide the loose hair at the back into three sections and plait each one, securing them with small, clear hair bands. (I,J)
8. Starting at the base, curl the plait loosely around itself and pin into place. (K,L)
9. Repeat this process for the other two plaits. Circle and figure-of-eight placements look nice, but there is no particular pattern to pinning them, so don't worry about them being perfect. (M)
10. Hide the ends by tucking them away and gripping them. (N)

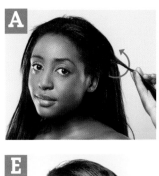

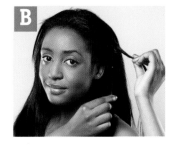

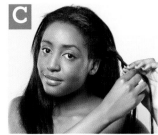

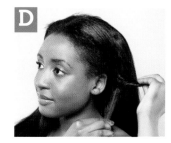

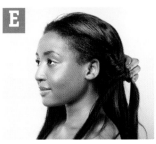

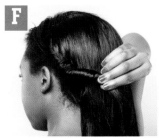

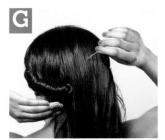

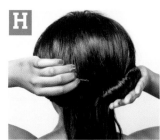

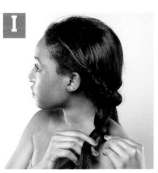

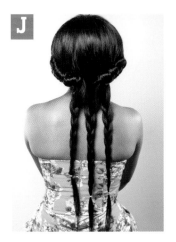

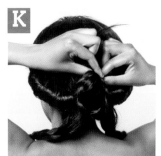

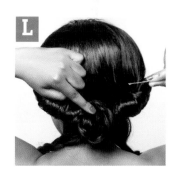

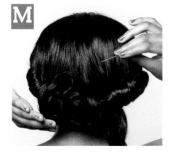

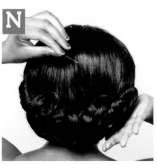

TIP

My hair is very fine: This style can lend itself to the use of some clip-in extensions. These can be used at the back to create thicker plaits, but not on the rolled side sections. Before you start rolling the hair, place one or two extension wefts horizontally at the centre of the back of the head. Make sure they are only 2/3 clip width wefts as they may become visible when rolling the sides if they are any wider. Pull your own hair down over the wefts to cover them and follow the instructions from the beginning.

To make the rolls look thicker, try not to pull them too tight, but do keep a firm grip on the hair and don't let it unravel. Once you get to the back of the head, holding the roll flat against your head, gently push it back towards the face. This will add a bit of extra volume to the roll.

My hair is very thick: Use extra-large hairpins to anchor the roll to your head. Fine pins may not be strong enough to control your hair.

Charm School

This is a fresh and pretty daytime look. The hair has a loose feel, whilst being twisted away from the face in a soft, sculpted curl. This style works with all hair types, including shorter hair so long as it can be gathered together or pinned up at the back. Flowers have been added to a large barrette to finish off the style.

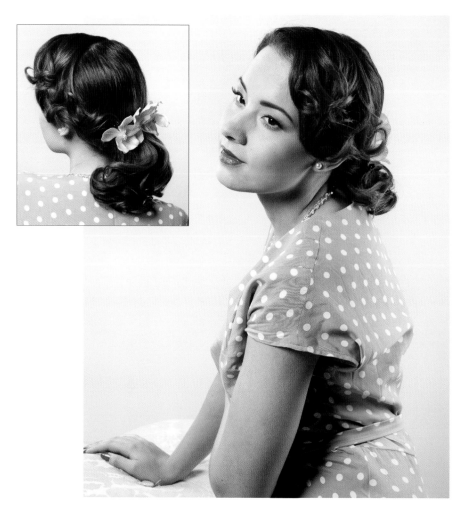

TECHNIQUES USED
Sculpted curls
Hot sticks

KIT LIST
Hot sticks (0.5 in/13mm)
Bristle brush
Tail comb
Pomade
Hairspray
Hairpins
Kirby grips
Banana clip/long barrette

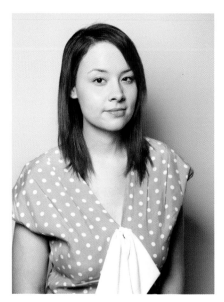

Shown on model with medium-length hair

Directions

1. Divide the hair into three sections. Make an ear-to-ear parting, with the hair at the front parted above the arch of the right eyebrow. (A,B)
2. Set the back of the head in hot sticks, rolling under. Roll the bottom half on base and the higher rows off base, leaving a large gap between the crown and the highest row of hot sticks. The front of the head is also set off base. (C,D,E)
3. Unwind the hot sticks, brush through the curls at the back of the head and gather into a loose ponytail. Secure the hair in place using a banana clip. Smooth and separate the curls in the ponytail into a loose, sculpted curl. (F,G)
4. Remove the remaining hot sticks and separate using pomade on your fingertips. If your hair is really curly, brush through the curls to loosen them before separating them with your fingers. (H)
5. Loosely twist the sections of hair away from your face and secure the curls in place, gripping any long sections to meet the ponytail at the back. (I,J)
6. On the opposite side, brush through the curls, gently twist the hair away from the face and grip into place. (K)

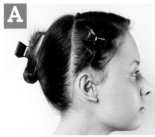

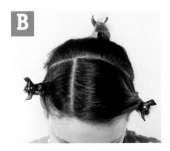

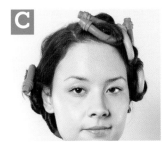

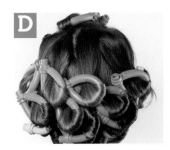

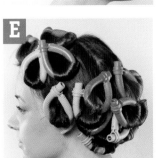

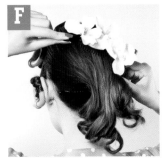

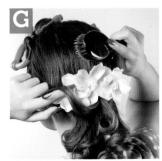

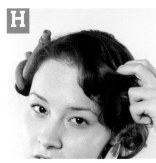

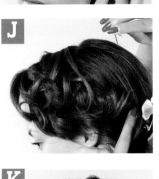

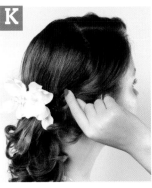

TIP

Alternative curling method: A small roller or tong would work for a hot set, and sponge, Velcro rollers or pin curls for a wet set.

My hair is very curly: A soft curl is required for the ponytail. If your hair has a tendency to hold curl really well, set the back hair in larger sections to obtain a looser curl. Alternatively, you could use a medium hot roller.

My hair is very long: You may need to support the ponytail at the back to prevent the curls from dropping. To maintain the short silhouette, loosely grip sections of the ponytail to give the illusion of a shorter length. Alternatively, leave the curls long and loose.

The Classic Snood

This charming wartime style is perfect when accessorized with a snood or scarf. Although heat is used, it could be attempted without if you leave the back straight and tucked into the snood, making it perfect for creating pin-up hair in a hurry. Alternatively, the style makes a great second- or third-day style following a previous pincurl set when there is still a bit of bend in the hair. The detail of the pin curl resting on the roll gives the style an added feature.

TECHNIQUES USED
Victory Rolls
Barrel Rolls

KIT LIST
Hot rollers (0.75 and 1in)
Hairgrips
Hairpins
Tail comb
Bristle brush
Pomade
Hairspray
Snood (optional)

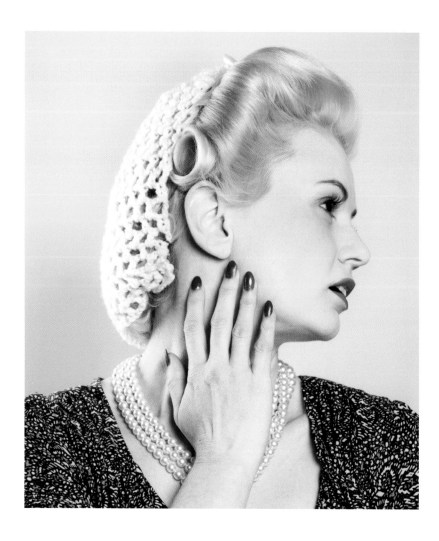

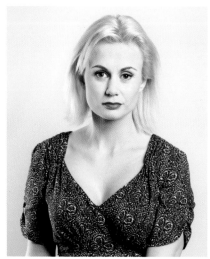

Shown on a model with medium-length hair.

Directions

1. Section your hair in an ear-to-ear parting. Set the front section in large rollers, on base, rolling away from the face. (A)
2. Set the back section of the hair in small rollers; the bottom half is set on base and the top half set off base, all rolling under. (B)
3. Leave to cool completely.
4. Back-brush the crown section thoroughly and smooth the top section of hair, ready for rolling. (C)
5. Form this section into a large Barrel Roll and secure with grips. (D,E)
6. Repeat the process on the lower section, pinning it up to meet the other roll in a Victory Roll. (F)
7. Use hairpins to gently join the two rolls and close any gaps. (G)
8. Repeat on the opposite side, forming one smaller Victory Roll. (H)
9. Use a tail comb to make any adjustments to the rolls. (I)
10. Use your fingers and some pomade to separate the hair at the back into fluff curls. (J)
11. Add a snood or scarf. Alternatively, omit the snood and just wear your curls loose.
12. Form one of the curls into a dry pin curl and pin to the base of the large Victory Roll. (K)

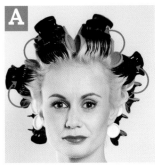

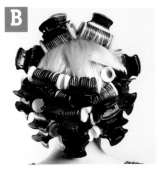

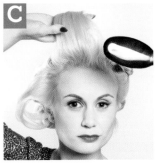

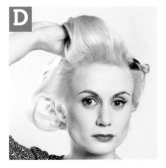

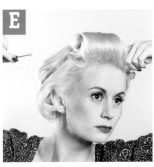

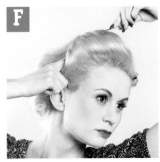

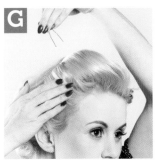

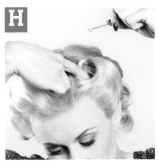

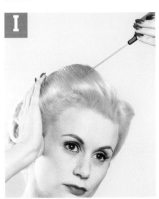

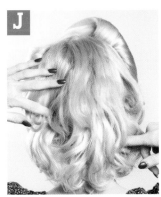

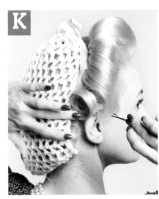

TIP

Alternative curling methods: Hot sticks, small tongs, pin curls, rag curls or wet rollers could be used to curl the back section. The front section could be curled using large tongs or elevated pin curls.

I have large gaps between my rolls: Try the hairpin technique to join the rolls.

My rolls do not cover the parting behind: Make the rolls larger and anchor them over the parting using hairpins.

In The Navy

This look features a braided hairpiece with the hair tucked around it in smooth rolls. The back is decorated with sculpted pin curls, which create a stylish feature at the rear of the style. This style works well for all hair types and is perfect for hair that struggles to hold curl as it is very secure.

See the 'Completing the Look' chapter for instructions on how to make your own hairpiece.

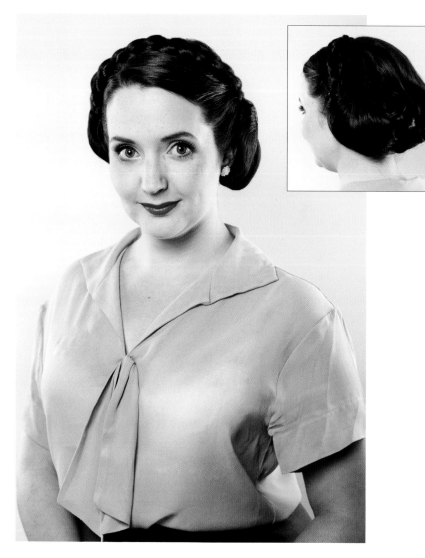

TECHNIQUES USED

Hot sticks

Pin curls (dry)

How to make a braided hairpiece: rope braid

KIT LIST

Hot sticks (0.5 in/13mm)

Bristle brush

Braided hairpiece

Pomade

Hairspray

Grips

Hairpiece

Combs

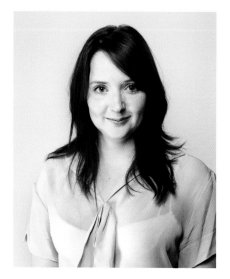

Shown on a model with long hair.

Directions

1. Set the hair in hot sticks, rolling under. All are set off base. Leave to cool completely. (A,B)
2. Remove the hot sticks and section the hair from ear to ear. (C)
3. Smooth back the first side section. (If you have very fine hair, you may want to add a bit of back-brushing for volume beforehand). (D)
4. Secure the side with a comb or grips. (E)
5. Work the hair towards your face into one smooth barrel curl, brushing the hair onto and around your hand. (F)
6. Repeat the process on the right side of the head.
7. Part the back of your hair into two even horizontal sections. Add stuffing or a rat in between the two sections and secure it with grips. (G,H)
8. Bring up sections of hair to cover and spread over the rat. (I)
9. Mist with hairspray and smooth any flyaway hairs upwards. (J)
10. Form the hair above the roll into rows of dry pin curls, gripping them

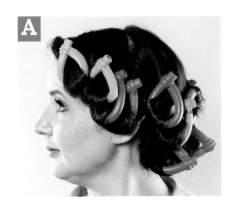

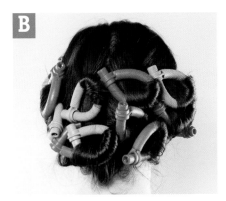

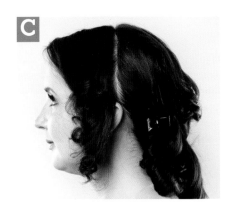

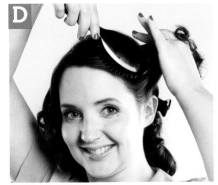

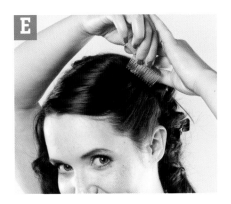

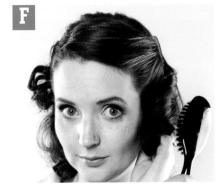

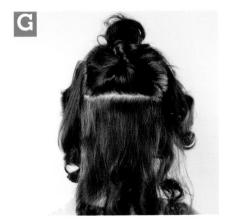

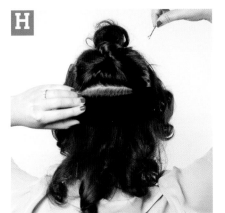

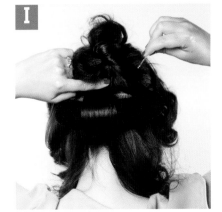

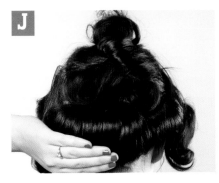

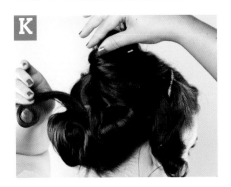

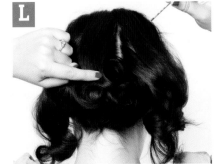

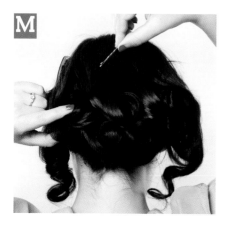

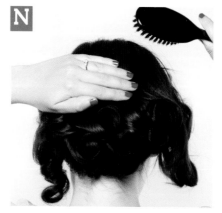

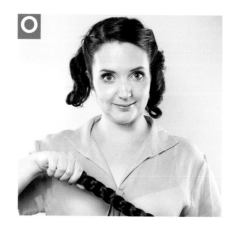

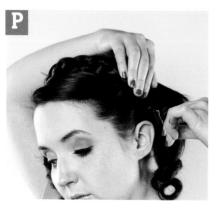

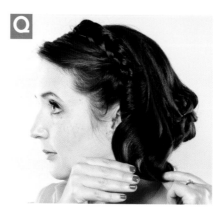

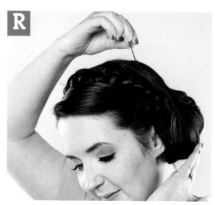

securely to the roll. Shape them around your fingers and roll to the head with the same method as a wet pin curl. (K,L,M)

11. Gently smooth the crown area, removing any gaps in the hair. (N)

12. Take a braided hairpiece and pin each end under the barrel curl on both sides of the head. (O,P)

13. Spread the barrel curl gently with your fingertips and pin it over the end of the hairpiece. (Q,R)

14. Repeat the process on the opposite side.

TIP

Alternative curling methods: You could set the hair in small rollers or a narrow-barrelled tong. A medium Velcro or sponge roller or pin curl would be the best choice for wet setting.

The Gibson Roll

The Gibson Roll or Gibson Tuck was fashionable during the Edwardian era, and made a comeback in the 1940s. The Gibson Roll or Tuck is an elegant up-style in which the hair is rolled over itself in a continuous reverse roll around the back of the head.

Dividing the hair into sections rather than attempting to roll it all at once makes the style easier to achieve. The fluffy curls are an interesting contrast to the sleek roll at the back of the head.

TECHNIQUES REQUIRED

Fluff curls

Victory Rolls

Blending with hairpins

Hot sticks

KIT LIST

Hot sticks (0.5 inch)

Hairpins

Kirby grips

Pomade

Hairspray

Hair rat

Bristle brush

Hair comb

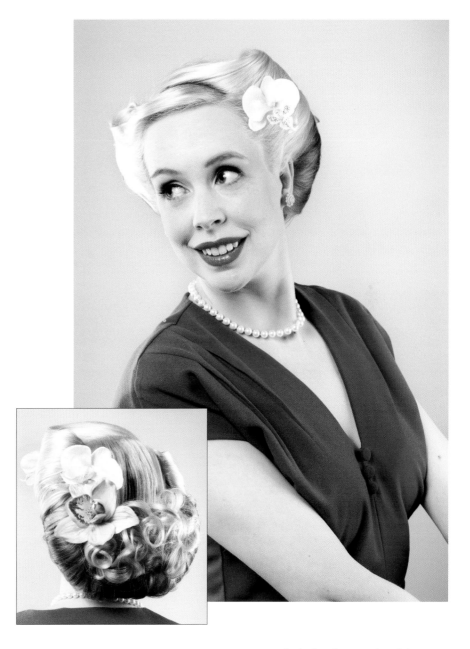

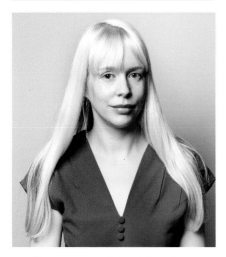

Shown on a model with long hair.

Directions

1. Make a parting from ear to ear. Divide this section into two above the arch of the right eyebrow and clip out of the way. (A,B)

2. Take a section a couple of centimetres wide at the top of the back section. Set this section off base in hot sticks. Take an extra-large synthetic doughnut, cut it so it forms one long section and pin it to the back of the head in a crescent shape (you can use two doughnuts pinned next to each other) and fix securely with grips. (C)

3. Divide the loose hair into three sections. Pull each section of hair up and over the doughnut, spreading the sections gently with your

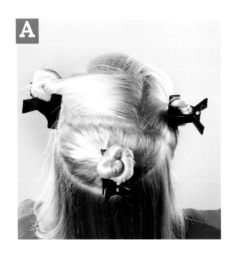

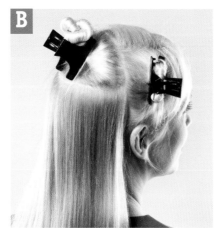

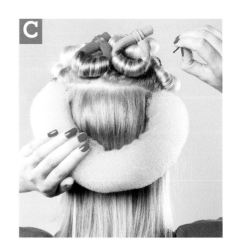

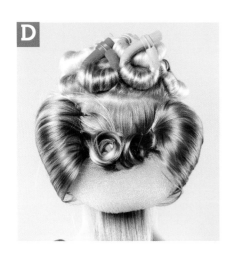

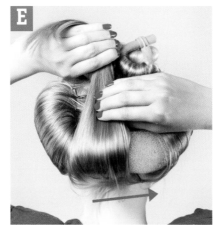

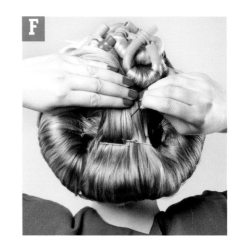

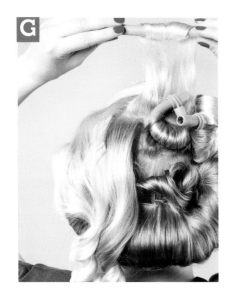

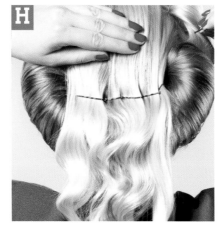

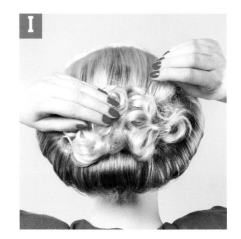

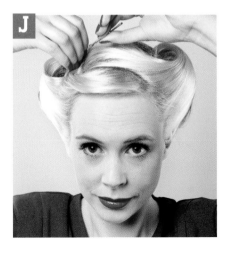

fingertips to cover the stuffing. Grip into place, pinning the ends into pin curls. Don't worry about the neatness of the pin curls as they won't be seen. (D,E,F)

4. Unwind the hot sticks. Smooth the hair and pull the whole section down to cover the pin curls so it meets the edge of the roll. Secure with grips. (G,H)

5. Pull the loose curls upwards and fix them into fluff curls, perching them on the ends of the roll and covering the grips. There is no pattern; just pin them randomly. (I)

6. Create a Victory Roll at each side of the head so that each roll meets the Gibson Roll at the back. Blend with hairpins to join the rolls if there are any gaps. (J)

7. If you have a fringe, pin it up to meet and blend with the rolls. If the hair is too straight to blend it, gently curl the fringe section before pinning.

Alternative curling methods: Set the hair in small rollers or tongs. A wet set with rollers or a pin curl set may also be used.

My hair is too silky to pin: This style works best on hair that hasn't been washed for 24–48 hours. If you find your hair is too silky to pin, tease it a little and apply some hairspray to give it some texture.

My hair is too short to cover the roll: Try clipping a couple of extension wefts at the base of your hairline at the back of your head. Use this hair to cover the roll, ensuring the roll sits low at the back of the head and covers the base of the hairline and the extension clips. Curl your shorter hair and sit the curls on top of the roll as per the instructions.

I cannot get the Victory Rolls and the Gibson Roll to meet: If blending the rolls with pins does not work, use decorated hairgrips, hair flowers or other accessories to conceal any gaps between the rolls.

My hair is very fine/thin: Use a smaller doughnut so there is not as much stuffing to cover. Back-brushing can be added to the top of the back section for more body.

Forces Sweetheart

This is a variation of the Gibson Roll. In this style no stuffing is used and the hair must be long enough to roll over itself at least once. The effect produces a smoother, shorter roll at the nape of the neck. This style also features Victory Rolls and a fringe roll, which is perfect if you like the look of rolls but do not like all of your hair pulled back completely off your face. This style looks stunning when accessorized with flowers or decorative combs.

TECHNIQUES USED

Victory Rolls
Barrel Rolls
Hot rollers
Blending with hairpins
Crossed grips

KIT LIST

Kirby grips
Hairpins
Hairspray
Pomade
Hot rollers (1/1.5 inch)
Tail comb
Bristle brush

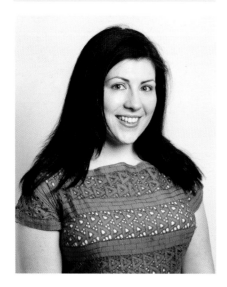

Shown on a model with long hair.

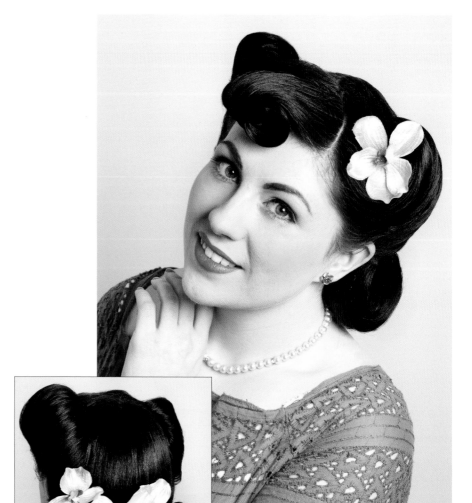

Directions

1. Set the whole head with large rollers (on base). This style can be done without pre-curling, but it is advisable if you find Victory Rolls tricky or have very fine hair. Leave the rollers to cool completely. (A)
2. Make an ear-to-ear parting. (B)
3. Smooth down the back section; a spritz of hairspray will help to control flyaway hairs and make the hair easier to manipulate. Secure with a line of crossed grips, holding firmly with one hand and pinning with the other. Make sure you pick up the lower layers of hair as well as the surface hair as you slide in the pins. (C)
4. Divide the back section into three and clip the two side sections up and out the way. (D)
5. Taking thin horizontal sections, back-brush the hair and roll into a horizontal Barrel Roll. Placing one finger inside the roll to secure, pin the roll into place. (E)
6. Repeat this step for the remaining

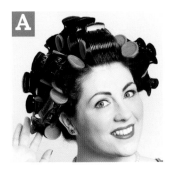

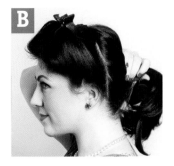

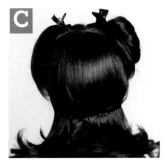

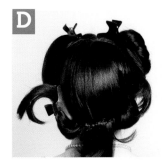

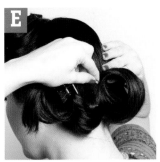

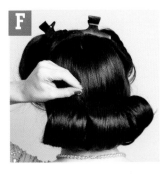

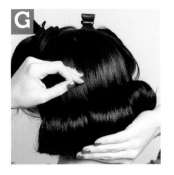

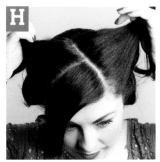

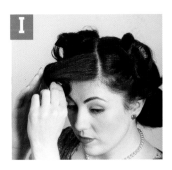

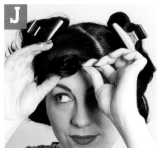

sections, trying to keep the rolls the same width and spreading the rolls gently with your fingertips to meet the first Barrel Roll in the centre. (F)

7. You may notice slight gaps between the rolls. Use hairpins to blend any gaps. (G)

8. Take a section at the front to be rolled into a fringe. Tease the fringe section thoroughly, smooth and roll into a Barrel Roll. Grip securely inside the roll. (H,I,J)

9. Roll the remaining two side sections into a Victory Roll on each side.

10. Finish the style with a mist of hairspray.

TIP

Alternative curling method: You can use a large-barrelled tong to set the hair, or use hot sticks on large sections to create a looser curl. You could also wet set the hair in large pin curls, Velcro or sponge rollers.

My hair is very fine: Before rolling the back section, clip a couple of extension wefts in horizontal sections, pulling the hair above down over the clips to blend them into the hair. This will provide more body in your roll and enable you to take larger sections at the front of the head to give the illusion of added thickness.

You could also push some crepe hair into the roll afterwards to bulk it out and close any gaps. Take care to grip it securely in place and make sure it is hidden well.

The Sophisticate

This upswept evening style is made up of a series of rolls that flow beautifully around the head. Pulling up the back section into a diagonal parting produces an interesting back feature.

This style works best on longer hair as sufficient length is required to be pulled to the top of the head and rolled over on itself at least once.

TECHNIQUES USED

Victory Rolls
Barrel Rolls
Hot rollers (0.75 and 1.25 in)
Crossed grips

KIT LIST

Kirby grips
Hairpins
Pomade
Hairspray
Tail comb
Bristle brush
Hot rollers

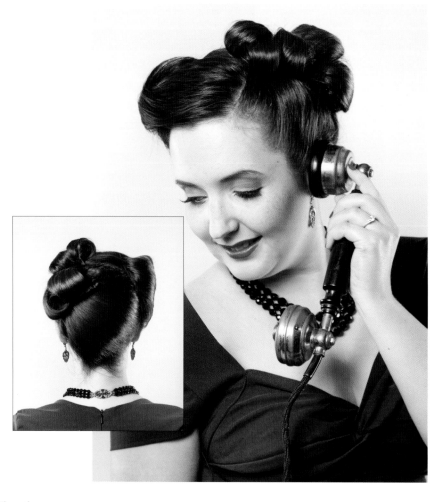

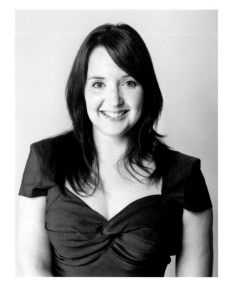

Shown on a model with long hair.

Directions

1. Divide the hair into three sections. Make an ear-to-ear parting and divide the front section in two above the arch of the left eyebrow. (A,B)
2. Set all the medium rollers at the back on base. Roll them upwards diagonally, in the same direction towards the left side of the head. (C)
3. The hair on the front left side of the head is also rolled at an upward slant around a small roller. These are set off base. The hair on the front right side of the head is set around medium rollers, rolled on base. (D)
4. Leave all of the rollers to cool completely.
5. Divide the back section in two and smooth the first section flat against your head in a diagonal direction. Secure with crossed grips. (E,F)
6. Repeat this with the lower section (this is done in two sections for ease). (G)
7. Take the loose ends of your hair and divide into two. Gently back-brush the first section and then smooth and roll it into a barrel curl. Repeat this process on the second section. (H,I,J)
8. Back-brush the large section on the right side of the head and smooth into a large Victory Roll. (K)
9. Taking the remaining section of hair, add a small amount of teasing at the

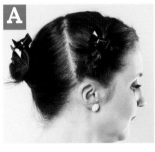

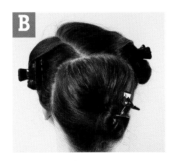

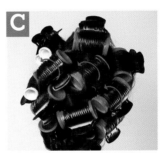

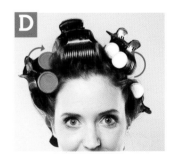

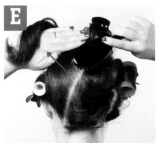

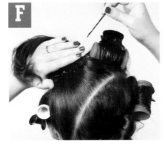

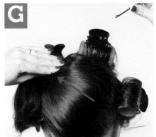

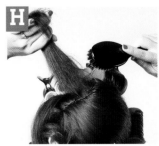

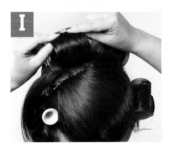

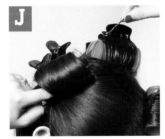

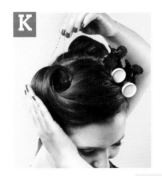

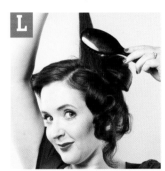

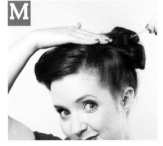

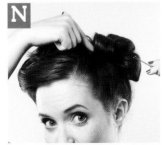

roots and smooth the hair diagonally upwards towards the crown. (L)

10. Secure with crossed pins. (M)

11. Taking the loose ends of remaining hair, form a few small Barrel Rolls in different directions, arranging them to meet the two rolls previously made at the back of the head. (N)

12. Mist the style with hairspray, smoothing any stray hairs on the rolls and around the hairline.

TIP

Alternative curling methods: A large- and small-barrelled tong can be used to set the hair. If you would like to wet set, use large and small Velcro or sponge rollers.

My hair is very thick: For ease of control, divide the hair into more Barrel Rolls.

My hair is very fine and my barrel curls are too skimpy: You could clip in a couple of single or double clip extensions and use them to make the barrel curls. Ensure you cover the clips by rolling the barrel curls outwards over the clips and spreading the curl to cover the sides of the clips.

Lovely Lucille

Lots of structured curls comprise this beautiful up style. This look is a perfect evening style for short hair, but it can also be recreated on long hair. Add combs adorned with flowers to match your outfit or, alternatively, add some sparkle for a special occasion.

TECHNIQUES REQUIRED

Hot sticks
Sculpted curls

KIT LIST

Hot sticks (0.5 inch)
Tail comb
Bristle brush
Pomade
Hairspray
Hairpins
Kirby grips
Combs

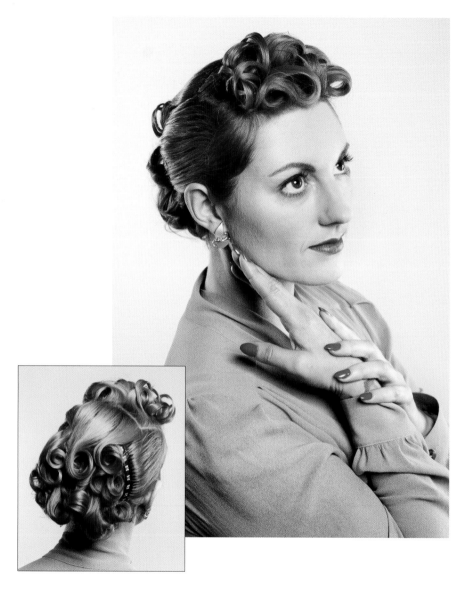

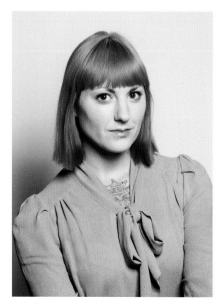

Shown on a model with short hair.

Directions

1. Section the hair with an ear-to-ear parting, dividing the front section into three by parting the hair above the arch of each brow. (A,B)
2. Set all of the hair in hot sticks. Set the back section with the lower section on base and the top section off base. The front-centre section is set on base whilst the two side front sections are set off base. Allow to cool completely. (C)
3. Brush the side sections up and back, securing with combs. (D,E,F)
4. Smooth through the curls at the back, brushing them into sculpted curls and pinning them randomly into place; there is no fixed pattern. (G,H)
5. Repeat the process for the curls at the front, smoothing and pinning them randomly into sculpted curls.
6. Finish with a mist of hairspray. (I,J)

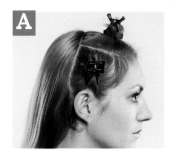

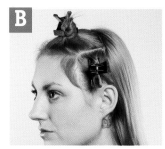

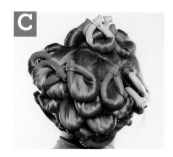

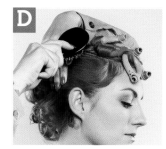

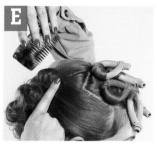

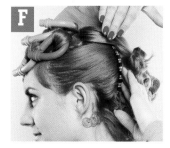

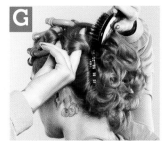

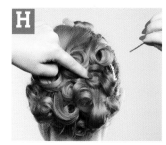

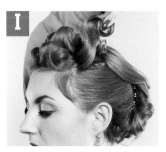

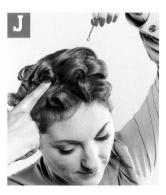

TIP

Alternative curling methods: Pin curls, rag rollers, small sponge or Velcro rollers all work well for this style. A small-barrelled tong would be the best option for a hot set.

My hair is very fine: For more volume and curl, clip some extension wefts at the back of the head, then style and blend with your own hair. Do not use pieces that are too wide as they will get in the way of the combs.

My hair is very thick: Section off an area of hair at the back in the middle of the curls. Twist this section to form a tightly coiled bun and grip to the head. This should remove some of the excess volume and provide a secure base on which to pin the curls.

Origami

This is a sleeker version of the Betty Grable style, with the main detail located at the back of the head. Based on a 1940s style called the Omelet Fold, the hair at the back folds inwards to create interesting detail.

TECHNIQUES USED

Crossed pins
Barrel Rolls
Sculpted curls

KIT LIST

Curling tongs (1.5 in)
Pomade
Hairpins
Hairgrips
Hairspray
Curl clips
Bristle brush

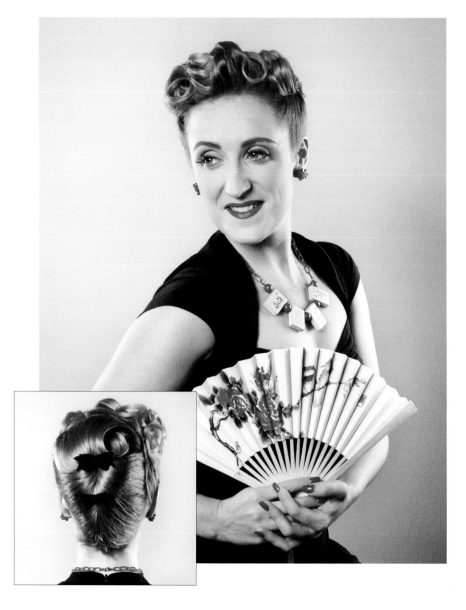

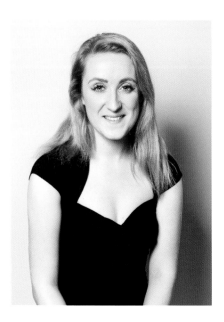

Shown on a model with long hair.

Directions

1. Make a parting from ear to ear. Divide the back section into three. (A,B)
2. Tong the top section horizontally with the curl rolling downwards. Roll the two lower sections vertically, rolling them both into the centre. The two lowest curls on each side roll upwards and the rest roll downwards in the same direction. (C)
3. Once all the curls have cooled completely, remove the two clips on the lower rolls at the back. Clip one side up and out of the way. Next, put horizontal layers of back-brushing through the other section. (D,E)
4. Brush the hair diagonally upwards to smooth the top layer and roll the section around two fingers into a barrel curl. Pull the hair taut diagonally, with the lower half of the

roll sitting tight against the head. If this isn't done, the rolls will have a baggy section below. Secure with a grip. (F,G,H)

5. Repeat the process on the opposite side so the rolls meet in the middle. (I)

6. Use hairpins to anchor the rolls in position and make any adjustments to the shape. (J)

7. Take the top of the back section and tease it in vertical sections. Smooth the top layer and roll into a vertical Barrel Roll. (K)

8. Gently spread the roll and place it so it sits nicely on the rolls beneath. (L,M)

9. Remove the curl clips at the front of the head. Smooth the side sections upwards and secure with crossed pins. (N)

10. Smooth the curls with pomade and pin them into sculpted curls, weaving them through each other for structure. There is no fixed pattern for pinning the curls. (O,P,Q)

11. Use a tail comb to make any adjustments or to add extra volume. (R)

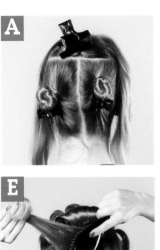
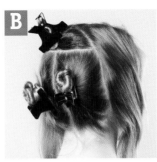
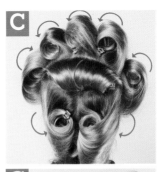
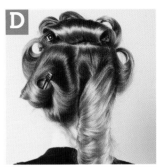
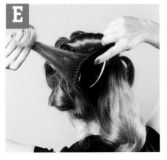
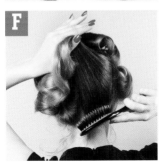
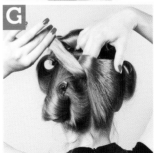
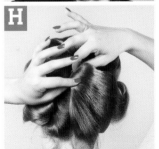
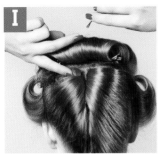
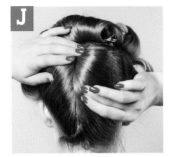
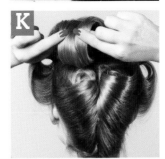
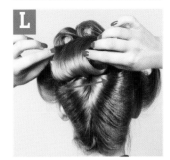

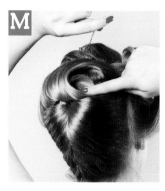

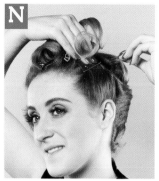

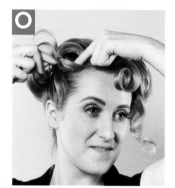

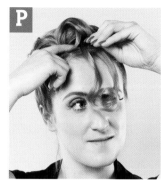

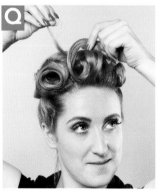

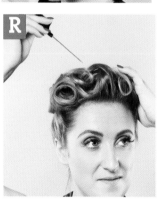

TIP

Alternative curling methods: If doing a wet set, large pin curls, sponge or Velcro rollers would work. If using heat, hot sticks are the best alternative.

I have fine hair/would like more volume: Separate the curls at the front section and create a base of crepe hair on which to pin the structured curls. This will provide more volume.

I don't like all my hair pulled back off my face: Allow a few of the curls to fall down onto your forehead, then pin the ends into position.

The Chignon Style

Hats were very popular in the 1940s; hence the popularity of smooth crowns, which feature in most styles of the era, as they create the perfect base for a hat. Lots of volume on the crown would cause the hat to sit at a funny angle.

The sleek crown and low chignon in this look work beautifully with a skull cap or tilt-style hat, which were very popular in the 1940s. This style is set on a long fringe, but could be adapted to cuts without a fringe.

TECHNIQUES USED

Shaping with clips
Curling tongs
Creating waves
Barrel Rolls

KIT LIST

Curling tongs (0.75 in)
Pomade
Hairspray
Hairgrips
Hairpins
Invisinet (optional)
Pin curl clip/duck-billed clips
Hair elastic
Bristle brush
Tail comb

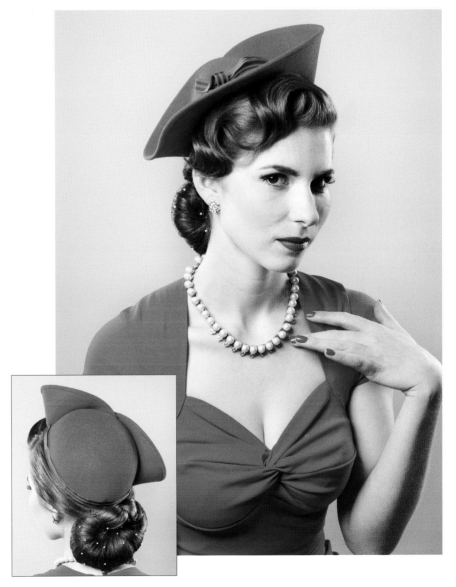

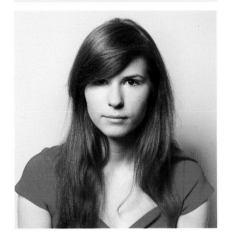

Shown on a model with long hair.

Directions

1. Pull the hair into a low ponytail, leaving the fringe section. If you have no fringe, section off a small section of hair at the front. (A,B)
2. Curl the front of the hair with tongs set at a diagonal, clipping the curls to allow them to cool. (C)
3. Part the hair directly above the ponytail to make a gap and push the ends of the ponytail up through the gap. This will create a twist in the hair. (D,E)
4. Smooth the hair above the ponytail. (F)
5. Taking horizontal sections, back-brush the ponytail and roll in to a Barrel Roll. (G,H)
6. Holding this in place securely with one hand, grip firmly inside the centre of the roll. (I,J)
7. Taking the edges in your fingertips, spread the roll upwards and outwards. (K)
8. Use pins to secure on either side. (L)
9. Give the chignon a thorough

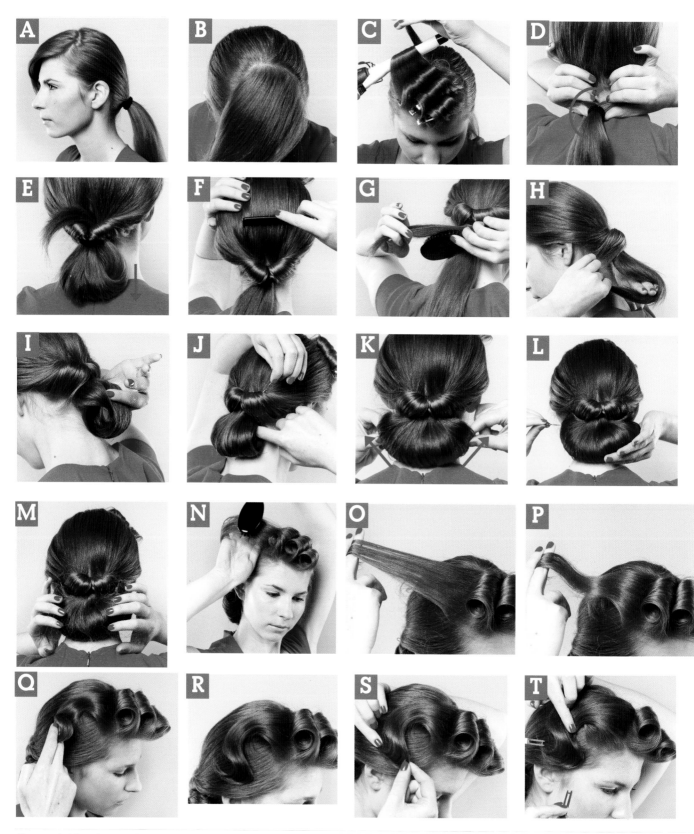

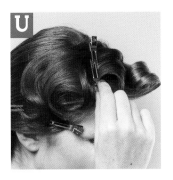
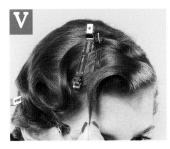
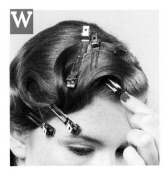
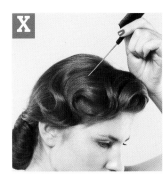

misting of hairspray and smooth with your hand or the end of a tail comb, tucking in any stray hairs. If there are any gaps, try blending with hairpins to join the chignon. You could add a fine net for extra support and to help push it together if any gaps remain. (M)

10. To style the hair on top of your head, starting with the bottom tube, remove the clip and brush through. Hold onto the end with your fingertips and release the tension on the hair to allow the wave to form. (N,O,P)

11. Lay the hair down onto the head, letting it sit in this natural wave. (Q,R)

12. When you are happy with how the wave is sitting, gently spread it with your fingertips and clip into place with curl clips. (S,T)

13. Repeat this process for subsequent sections, using the clips to shape your style and accentuate the waves. (U,V,W)

14. Apply a thorough mist of hairspray and let any tackiness dry before removing the clips.

15. Use a tail comb to make any adjustments and add volume if you wish. (X)

TIP

I don't have a fringe: You can still attempt this style. Make a parting as per the instructions and simply tuck the long ends of the hair under the chignon and grip into place once the wave is created.

I am finding the chignon tricky: Pre-curl the ponytail section before styling. This will give the hair some bend and make styling easier.

My hair is very straight and slippery: Add some back-combing spray or dry shampoo to the chignon before styling; this will make shaping the hair easier.

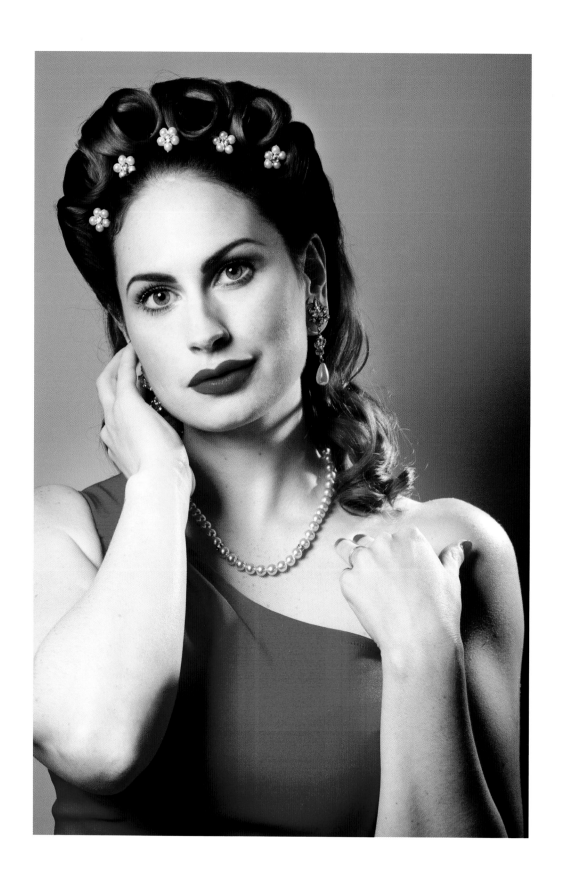

Chapter 7
Step-by-step Guide to Classic Down Styles

Short and Sweet

This cute and curly style works well on short hair, and the fluff curls provide volume to fine hair. With longer hair, the back could be pinned up loosely to recreate the short silhouette. This is a perfect daytime style.

The Faux Victory Rolls are perfect for vintage hair beginners, as they give the impression of a Victory Roll by simply pushing the side sections forwards.

TECHNIQUES USED
Fluff curls
Shaping with clips
Faux Victory Rolls

KIT LIST
Hot sticks (0.5 in)
Long curls clips
Pomade
Hairspray
Kirby grips
Hair comb/slide (optional)
Bristle brush
Tail comb

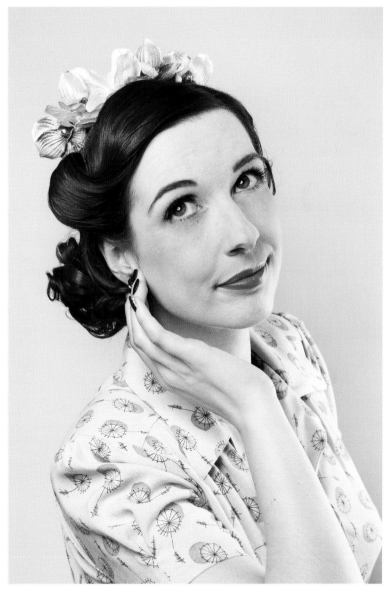

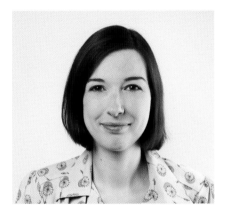

Shown on a model with short hair.

Directions

1. Make an ear-to-ear parting. Divide the front section into two. (A,B)
2. Set the hair in hot sticks. The hot sticks at the back are set on base at the bottom of the head and off base at the top. All the hot sticks at the front are on base. (C,D)
3. Leave the hot sticks to cool thoroughly.
4. Unwind the sticks from the back section and separate the hair into fluff curls. (E)
5. Smooth the crown section. (F)

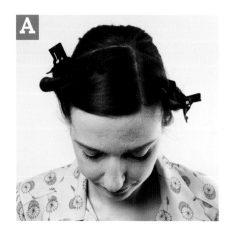

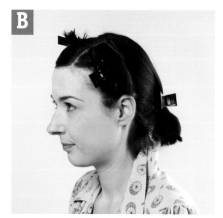

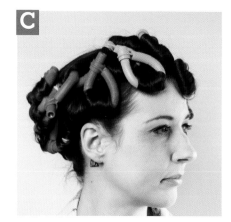

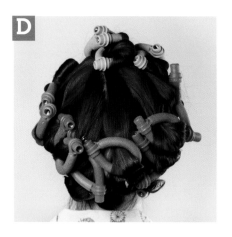

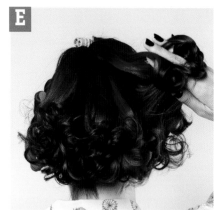

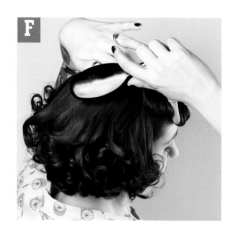

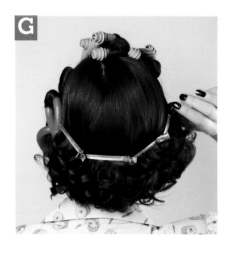

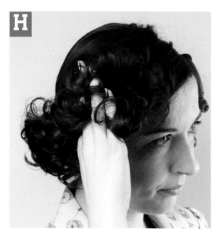

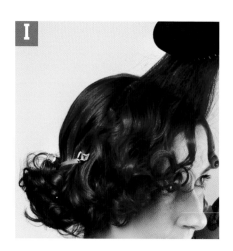

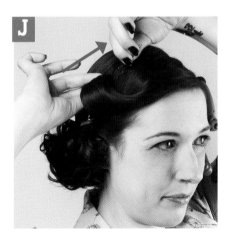

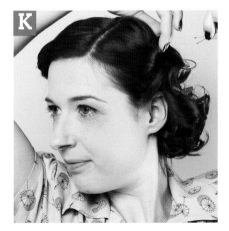

6. At the ridge of the curls at the back of your head, clip with duck-billed clips and add a mist of spray. This accentuates the halo effect you have created. (G)

7. Brush through the front section with your fingers to separate the curls. (H)

8. Lightly back-brush this section or mist it with dry shampoo or back-combing powder. Pinch the hair in your fingertips, pull the hair up and back and then push it forwards, creating a Faux Victory Roll. (I,J)

9. Smooth up the hair on the other side of your head and push it forwards, creating volume at the root. Secure with grips or a comb. (K)

10. Finish the style with a mist of hairspray.

TIP

Alternative curling methods: Use tongs or a wet set instead. Ensure the barrel, roller or pin curl is small enough to achieve a tight fluff curl. Rag curls would work well here.

My hair is very fine: Add some back-combing at the crown. You could bulk out the back section with some extension wefts, curling them with a small tong or clipping them in place and rolling with hot sticks. Brush out the hair in accordance with the instructions.

Hat Style

These rolls are designed to be worn with a 1940s saucer hat. The volume is all on one side of the style so the tilt hat sits perfectly on the flat side while the sculpted rolls are visible underneath. The model has long hair, but this style would work well on any length, providing it is sufficient to roll over on itself once.

If you wish to wear the style without a hat, skip the flat pin curls and style both sides into Victory Rolls.

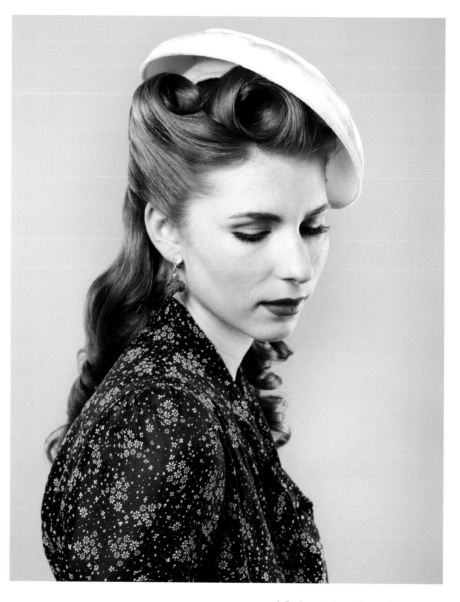

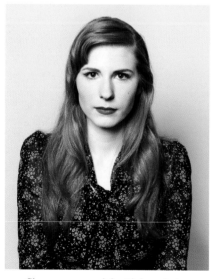

Shown on a model with long hair.

Directions

1. Divide the hair into four sections. Make a parting from ear to ear. Divide the hair in front of the ears into three sections. Take a diagonal parting above the arch of the right eyebrow and another from the arch of the left eyebrow, making a triangular section in the middle of the head. (A,B)

2. Curl these sections with a large-barrelled tong for volume and clip to cool. Both outside sections roll upwards and the middle section rolls down to meet the right-hand section. (C)

3. Tong the back of the head with a small-barrelled tong and clip to cool. The curls at the bottom are rolled on base, while the top section of curls is rolled off base with a smooth crown. (D,E)

4. Remove the clips from the back section and smooth the curls with pomade, brushing them around your

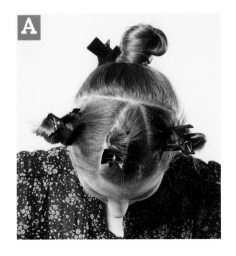

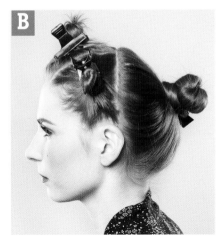

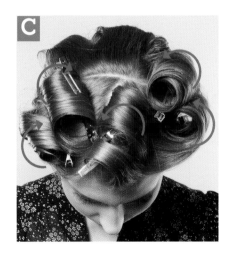

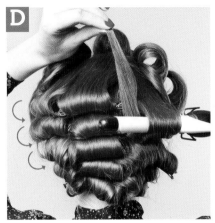

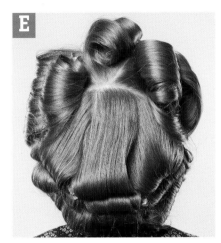

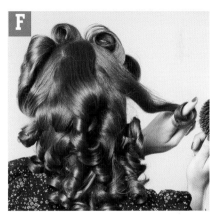

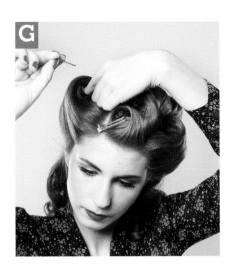

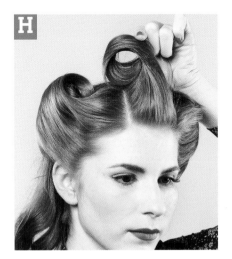

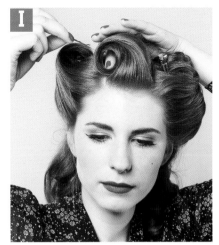

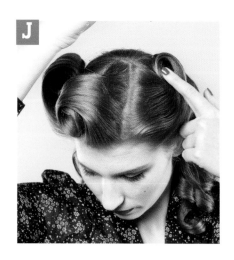

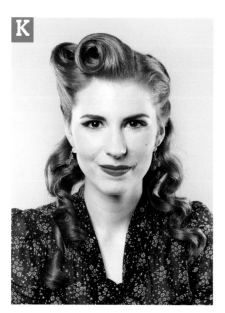

TIP

Alternative curling method: Use small sponges or Velcro rollers, rag or pin curls to recreate this look. If rag-rolling the front, ensure you use bigger sections as the curl shouldn't be too tight for the Victory Rolls. Hot sticks are a good heat option.

I have very fine hair: To add the illusion of thicker or longer hair, add a few extension wefts at the back of your head. However, ensure they are cut to your length so they blend easily. By doing so you could take a larger ear-to-ear section, bulking out the rolls at the front.

My hair is short: This style will work on shorter hair, providing there is sufficient length at the front to roll over on itself.

finger for a smooth, structured curl. (F)

5. Remove the clips at the front and back-brush the right-hand section thoroughly, rolling it into a large Victory Roll. (G)

6. Create another roll with the middle section, pinning it to cover the parting and meet the other Victory Roll. (H,I)

7. With the final section, roll the hair into a large, flat pin curl, adding a small amount of teasing. This will make a perfect base for a tilt hat. (J,K)

8. Set the style by applying a mist of hairspray, taking care to let the hair dry away any tackiness before putting on a hat.

The Smoothie

This style is a much softer version of the quintessential 1940s look, the Pageboy. This style is sleek all over with softly tucked ends and topped with a single pin curl at the front. The wet set will help to keep the brushed-out, smooth nature of this style from dropping.

This is the perfect style to brush your hair into a day or two after trying one of the tighter curled styles, such as Old Hollywood or the Lamarr. At this stage, your curls will have dropped and you will need a brush-through to tidy.

TECHNIQUES USED

Velcro rollers

Shaping with clips

Brushing into waves

Pin curls (dry)

KIT LIST

Velcro rollers (1 inch)

Setting lotion

Styling brush

Pomade

Kirby grips

Hair comb

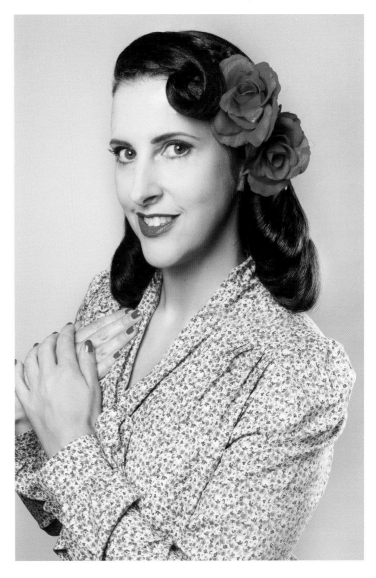

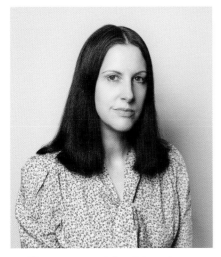

Shown on a model with long hair.

Directions

1. Section the hair into an ear-to-ear parting. (A,B)
2. Set the hair in Velcro rollers. The back section rolls under with the rollers set off base. The rollers at the front are also set slightly off base, rolling under towards the face. (C,D)
3. Wait until the set is completely dry and remove the rollers. Using pomade, brush out the hair, always brushing it over and under the hand. (E)
4. Use long curl clips to accentuate the natural ridge created by the smooth curl at the back of the head. Mist with hairspray and leave to dry. (F)
5. Pull back the hair at both sides of the head, and secure with a comb. This accentuates the beautiful barrel curls created on either side. (G)
6. Add a small amount of back-brushing to the front section, smoothing out the top layer of hair after teasing to give a smooth finish. (H)
7. Roll this section into a dry pin curl and secure. (I,J)

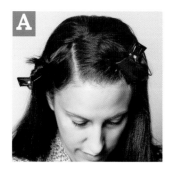

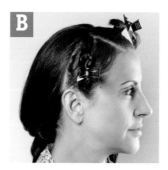

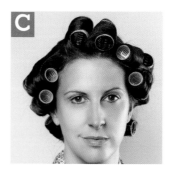

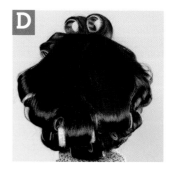

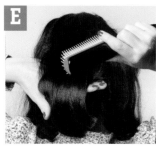

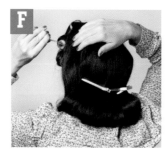

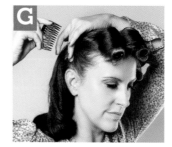

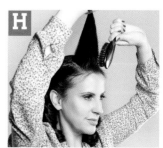

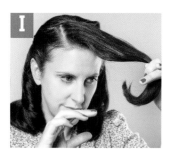

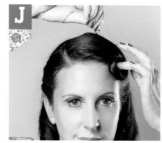

TIP

Alternative curling methods: If your hair curls very well, you could use hot rollers or tongs. You could also use a large pin curl, all set rolling towards the face.

My hair cannot hold the soft curl: This is a very difficult style to achieve for hair that doesn't always hold curls well as it has a tendency to drop. Remedy this by placing the hair in an ultra-fine 'invisinet' of matching colour, securing the net behind the dry pin curl and over the barrel curls on either side of the head. If you have hair that is resistant to curling, try setting it with a slightly thinner roller. This will give the curl more chance of holding following the brush-out.

My hair is very fine: You might want to add some back-brushing to the side sections before you secure them with the comb.

Half and Half

This look features fluff curls that contrast with smooth rolls and a beautiful wave at the back of the head. This style can be created on much short or long hair. As long as the hair is long enough to be formed into a Victory Roll, the look can be recreated.

Directions

1. Section the hair into four sections using a tail comb. Make a parting from ear to ear. Divide the section in front of the ears into three: one large

TECHNIQUES REQUIRED

Tongs
Hot sticks
Victory Rolls
Fluff curls
Brushing in to waves
Unified wave technique

KIT LIST

Tongs (1.5 inch)
Hot sticks (0.5 inch)
Bristle brush
Tail comb
Pomade
Hairspray
Grips
Combs

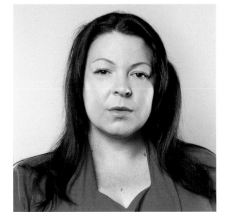

Shown on a model with long hair.

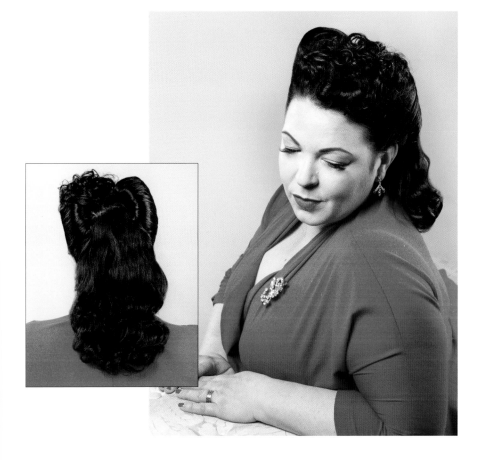

diagonal section on the right side of the head and two small diagonal sections on the left. (A,B)

2. Set the back section in hot sticks with an off-base crown. Set the centre-front section in hot sticks also; these are set on base and can be rolled in different directions with no set pattern. Make sure they are set in small sections to attain a very strong curl. (C)

3. Set the two side sections with a large tong and clip to cool. The aim here is to create volume rather than a strong curl. (D,E)

4. Leave the set to cool completely and remove the hot sticks from the back section of hair. Separate the hair with your fingers and some pomade. (F)

5. Brush through the hair with a styling brush, combining it into one smooth wave. (G,H)

6. Remove the curl clips and hot sticks from the front of the hair. First, take the largest outside section and back-brush it throughout. Smooth the top layer and roll it into a large Victory Roll, spreading it with your fingertips. (I,J)

7. Repeat the process on the opposite outside section. This roll will be slightly smaller. (K)

8. Using pomade, separate the central section into several small, defined fluff curls. Gently twist the curls around each other to hold them in place. (L)

9. Use hairpins to secure the style. This will help retain the loose look of the curls but provide some security. (M)

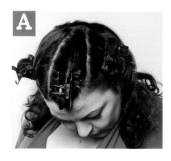

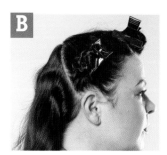

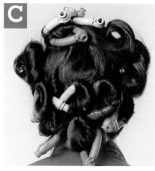

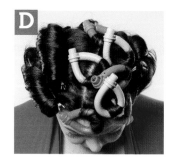

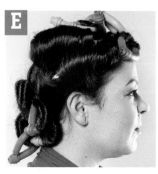

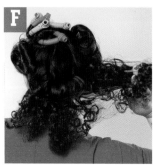

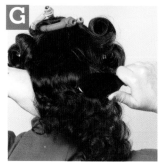

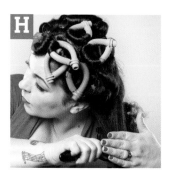

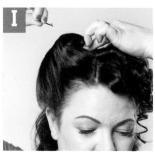

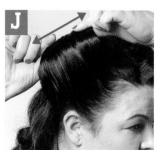

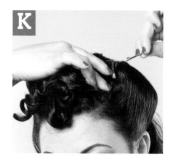

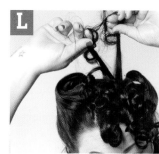

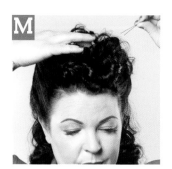

TIP

Alternative curling method: Pin curls would work for this style, along with small sponge or Velcro rollers. A small-barrelled tong would work well for the curls at the back and the fluff curls at the front. Use a wider tong to achieve a volume curl in the Victory Roll sections before rolling.

I don't like all my hair pulled back: If you prefer to have a fringe, let a few of the curls fall onto the forehead.

I have a fringe: Curl the hair using hot sticks or tongs as instructed. This will blend with the longer sections of hair behind.

The Crown

This regal style was inspired by the actress Ann Southern. The sculpted rolls resting on the sleek front section create a crown effect. The back section also features a sculpted curl with a smooth peak. To accentuate the tiara-like effect, the rolls can be accessorized with jewels and pearls on pins or clips.

TECHNIQUES USED

Barrel Rolls
Sculpted curls
Crossed grips
Hot rollers

KIT LIST

Hairpins
Kirby grips
Tail comb
Bristle brush
Hairspray
Pomade
Hot rollers (0.75 and 1 inch)

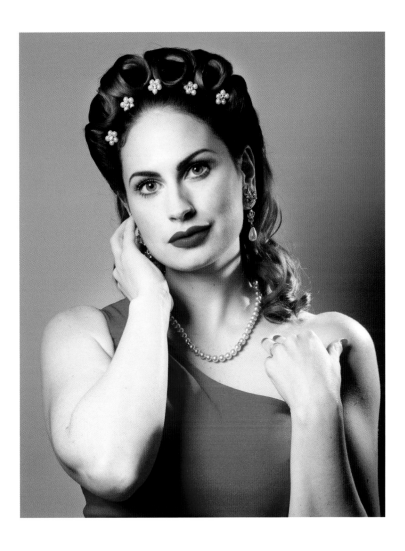

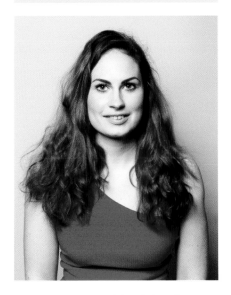

Shown on a model with long hair.

Directions

1. Divide the hair in to four sections. Make an ear-to-ear parting. Next, divide the front section into three, making two partings above the arch of each of the brows. (A)

2. Set the hair in rollers all rolling under. Use a small roller at the back to form a defined curl and a larger roller at the front for volume and bend. Set the rollers at the front on base. The rollers at the back are set on base in the lower half of the head and off base in the top half, producing volume with a smooth crown. (B,C)

3. Remove the rollers, smooth the central crown section and secure with cross pins. (D)

4. Back-brush one side, form it into a Victory Roll and secure. (E)

5. Repeat this process on the opposite side. (F)

6. The central section will now be rolled into four separate Barrel Rolls on top of the head. Divide the hair into four equal sections. Take the first section and roll it into a Barrel Roll, sitting at a diagonal. Use your fingers to spread the hair and accentuate the off-centre direction of the roll you have created. Secure

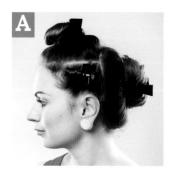 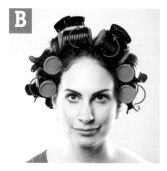 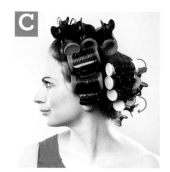 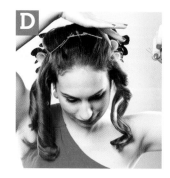

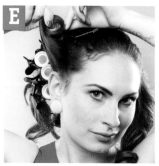 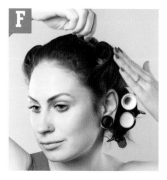 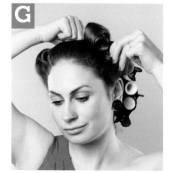 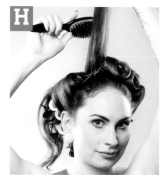

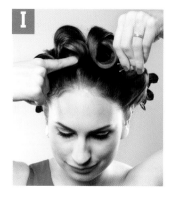 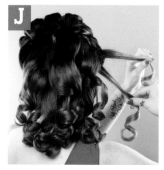 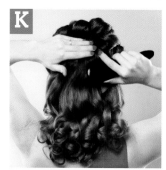

with a grip inside the roll and anchor with a hairpin at the back of the roll. (G)

7. Repeat this process for the three remaining sections. (H,I)

8. Remove the rollers from section four and separate into sculpted curls. (J)

9. Smooth the crown section and brush with a light mist of hairspray. (K)

10. Finish the style with a mist of hairspray.

TIP

Alternative curling methods: If your hair is resistant to curling, try a different method to set the curls, for example tongs. Alternatively, try a wet set with sponge/Velcro rollers or pin curls.

You can see through my crown rolls: Try forming the rolls in more of a diagonal shape. Anchor down the roll at the back with a hairpin.

Old Hollywood

Rita Hayworth's tumbling waves made her a true hair icon. This classic Old Hollywood style worn by Rita in *Gilda* features soft, flowing waves and a smooth, sleek crown, with the bulk of the wave sitting at the bottom of the hair.

The soft layers through the model's hair allow the curls to sit in a smooth waterfall effect. These bombshell waves will take you from day to night and are perfect for a glamorous evening out.

TECHNIQUES USED

Pin curls

Brushing into waves

Shaping with clips

KIT LIST

Pin curl clips

Duck-billed clips

Styling brush

Hairspray

Pomade

Styling brush

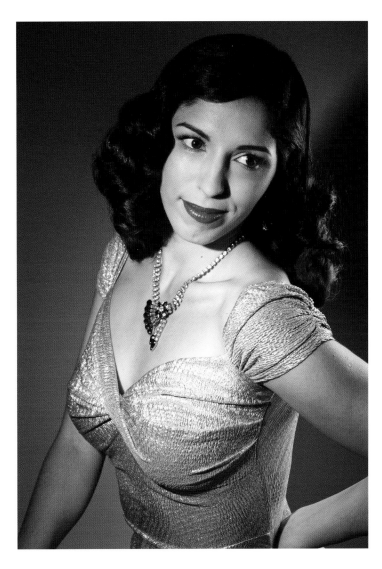

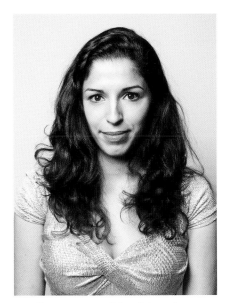

Shown on a model with long hair.

Directions

1. Set the hair in medium pin curls, following the specific pin curl pattern for this style. (A)
2. Coat your fingertips with a small amount of pomade and gently separate the curls. (B)
3. Start brushing through your hair with a styling brush, brushing the hair in to waves. (C)
4. Keep brushing the hair until the wave sits at the bottom of the hair and the hair begins to mould into one. A mist of hairspray will help mould the hair as you work. (D)
5. Use clips to accentuate the wave forming at the front of the hair. (E)
6. Keep brushing until you are happy with the finish and the frizz has been removed. (F)
7. You can gently lengthen and accentuate these waves by spreading the hair with your fingertips. (G,H)
8. Smooth any stray hairs with pomade and use your hands to smooth and sculpt the waves you have created. (I)
9. Finish the style with a mist of hairspray.

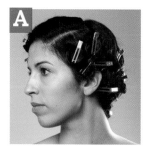

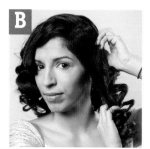

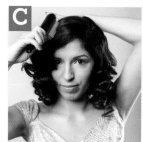

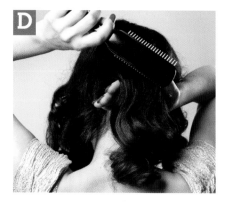

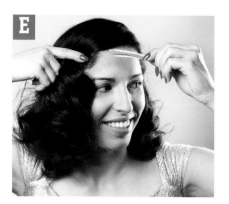

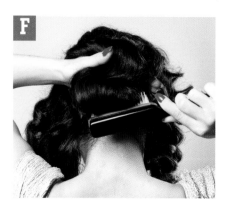

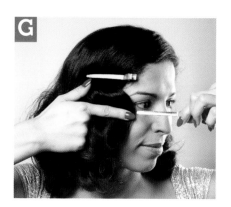

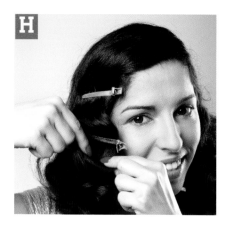

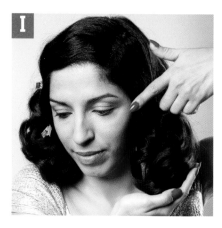

Sweeping Pompadour

This pompadour creates a curved, sweeping shape rather than just a straight tube, due to the mix of large and small pin curls in the setting pattern. The hair needs to be long enough to be rolled over on itself as least once, but the hair at the back can be much shorter; and as long as it can be curled, any length is fine for this style.

TECHNIQUES REQUIRED

Elevated pin curls
Unified wave
Foam rollers
Fluff curls
Barrel Rolls

KIT LIST

Foam rollers (0.75 inch)
Styling brush
Bristle brush
Kirby grips
Pin curl clips
Setting lotion
Hair combs

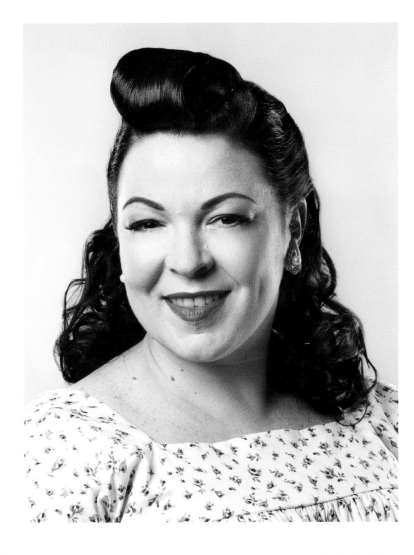

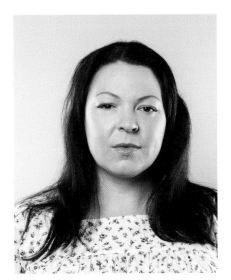

Shown on a model with long hair.

Directions

1. Section off a large section at the front of the head. This starts above the arch of each brow and back to the crown of the head, getting thinner as you get to the crown. (A)
2. Set the sides and back of the hair in foam rollers, leaving the crown off base. (B)
3. The elevated pin curls are set in three rows. The middle row is set in medium pin curls, while the two outer rows are set in small pin curls. All the pin curls roll forwards towards the face. (C)
4. Once the hair is completely dry, separate the curls in to fluff curls. (D)
5. Smooth the side sections of hair up with a bristle brush and secure with combs. (E)
6. Separate the front section using pomade and brush through. Tease the hair at the roots. (F)
7. Place your hand in the hair, positioning it to sit as far back as the parting on the crown. (G)
8. Smooth the top layer of hair over your hand and roll into a large Barrel Roll. (H,I)
9. Seat the hair on the head and gently spread the edges of the roll with your fingertips; the edges will

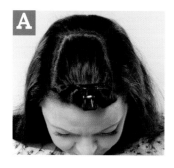

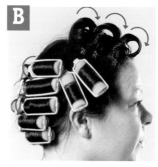

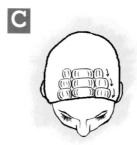

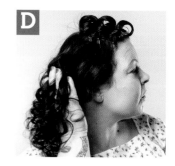

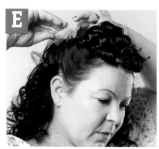

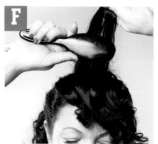

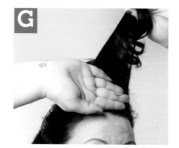

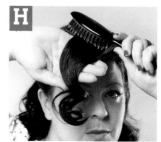

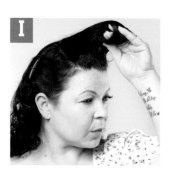

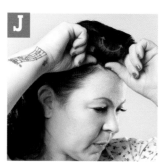

naturally curl upwards, creating a
curved roll. (J)

10. Secure with grips.

11. Apply a mist of hairspray to set the
style.

TIP

Alternative curling method: Small pin
curls or rags could be used for the fluff
curls at the back of the head. The best
heat method for the front would be tongs
as precision curls of two different sizes are
needed to set the front section.

My hair is fine/thin: Add volume at the
sides by back-brushing before you fix with
combs. Wefts could be added for extra
volume at the back, curling and blending
them with your own hair.

My hair is thick: If your hair is very
thick, take a slightly smaller section for
the pompadour. Keep the width of the
parting the same but remove some of the
hair from the back of the section before
setting. This will make it easier to handle.

The Bad Girl

This seductive style is inspired by the first lady of film noir, Veronica Lake. The front sits close to the head in an S-shaped wave, whilst the loose curls at the ends of the hair fall softly around the shoulders, leaving a smooth and sleek crown. The wave at the front of the head is known as a shadow wave, which is a soft finger wave with no ridges.

TECHNIQUES USED

Shadow waves

Pin curls

KIT LIST

Setting lotion

Styling comb

Gel (optional)

Pin curl clips

Duck-billed clips

Styling brush

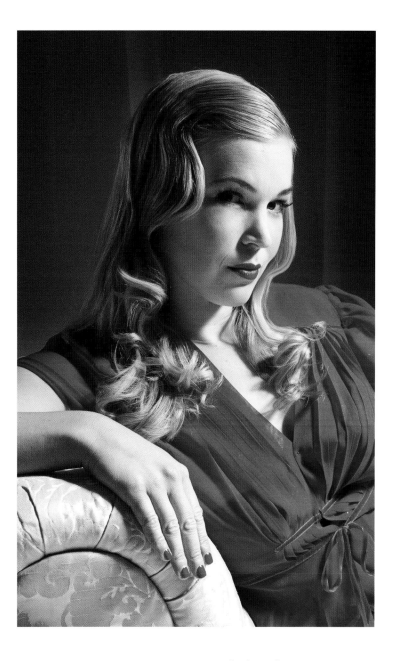

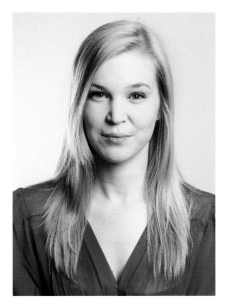

Shown on a model with long hair.

Directions

1. Make a deep parting in the hair. (A)
2. Dampen the front section of the hair with water and a firm-hold setting lotion or gel, ensuring the hair is sufficiently wet. Brush the hair diagonally away from the face, making sure the teeth of the comb make contact with your scalp. (B)
3. Hold this section of hair flat with your index finger, keeping pressure on the hair and holding it securely at all times. (C)
4. Use a long curl clip to hold this section in place. (D)
5. Place your index finger over the clip and hold the hair securely in place. Comb the hair towards the face in the opposite direction to the first section. Once again, do this in a

firm action so that the comb connects with your scalp. (E)

6. Secure this section with a clip. (F)

7. Repeat this process, changing direction and combing towards the back of the head. As before, hold the previous section in place securely as you comb. (G)

8. Secure with another clip. (H)

9. You can now remove the middle clip. (I)

10. Set the rest of the head in large pin curls, around two or three fingers in width. These are off base and should not go any higher than the nape of the neck. (J)

11. Ensure the set dries fully before proceeding to the next step. You may need a hood dryer as the front of the hair can take a while to dry.

12. Remove all of the clips. Brush through the wave at the front of the head with a styling brush. (K)

13. Replace the two long curl clips holding the S-wave at the front of the head and mist it with spray. This will hold the wave in place as you brush out the rest of the curls. (L)

14. Add some pomade and gently brush out the waves at the ends of your hair. This is a very loose, undefined wave, with just a hint of curl at the ends. (M)

15. Remove the long curl clips and set the style with a mist of hairspray. Secure with a pin if necessary.

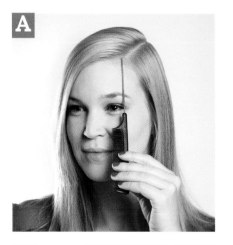

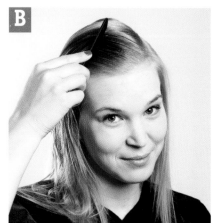

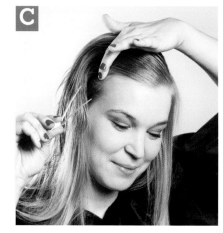

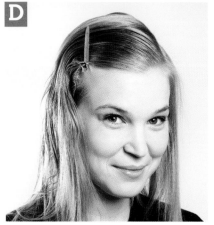

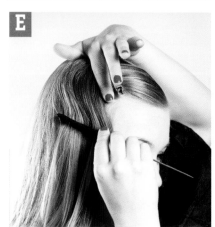

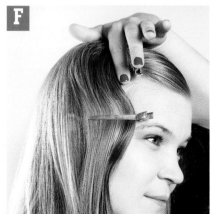

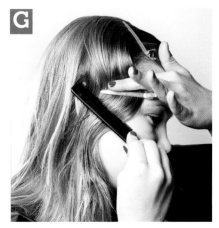

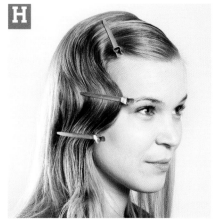

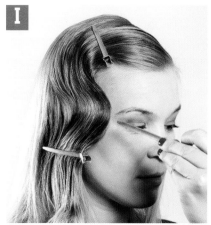

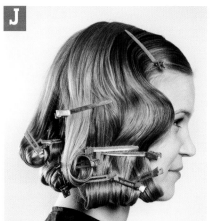

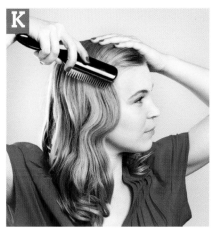

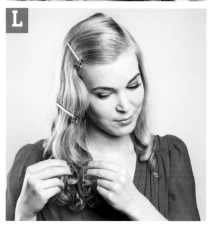

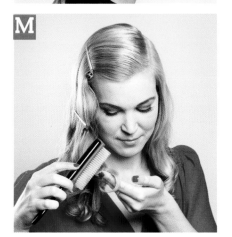

TIP

Alternative curling methods: A medium sponge or Velcro roller could be used at the back of the head, or a medium-barrelled tong or hot roller if heat is used.

My hair is very thick: Try using a wider-toothed comb to comb in the waves at the front section waves, as it will move more easily through the hair.

My hair drops easily: Use a decorative clip to hold the bottom of the S-wave in shape to prevent the hair losing its shape.

Cocktail Lounge

This seductive hairstyle features a large, sculpted S-wave with defined curls, swept dramatically to one side. Although the model has long hair, this style also works on much shorter hair. Accessorize the look with bright flowers or a jewelled comb to add eye-catching elegance

TECHNIQUES USED

Pin curls
S-wave
Sculpted curls

KIT LIST

Curl clips
Tail comb
Duck-billed clips
Setting lotion
Styling brush
Kirby grips
Hairspray
Pomade

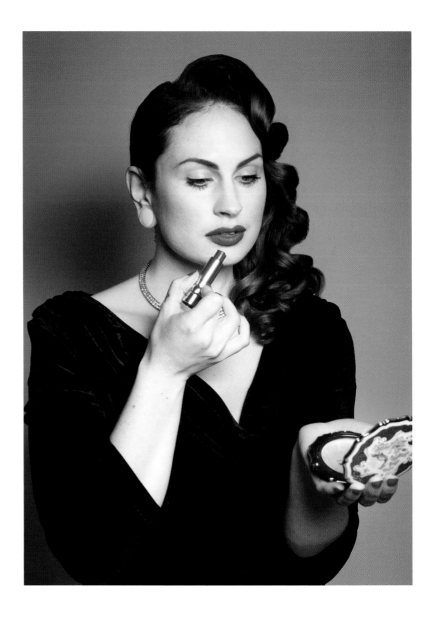

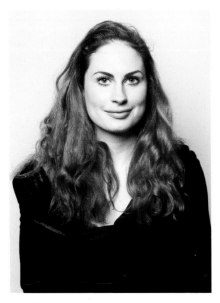

Shown on a model with long hair.

Directions

1. Set the entire head in medium pin curls following the pin curl pattern for this style. The elevated pin curls all roll towards the face and the rest of the hair is set in alternating rows. Ensure they have dried thoroughly before removing the clips. (A,B)

2. Remove the pins and separate the curls using your fingers and a small amount of pomade. (C)

3. Using a styling brush, brush through the crown section. (D)

4. Next back-brush this section thoroughly with a bristle brush, adding hairspray as you go. (E)

5. Smooth the top layer of hair. (F)

6. Place your finger into the hair as a support on which to brush the wave and create the first bend of the S. (G,H)

7. Use duck-billed clips to help shape the wave. (I)

8. Use your fingers to gently spread the

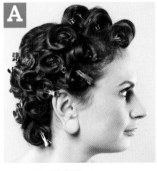

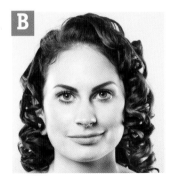

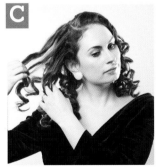

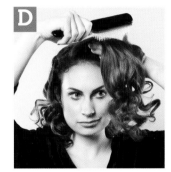

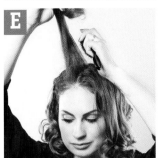

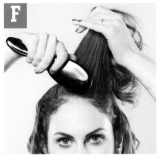

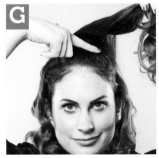

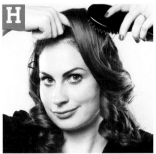

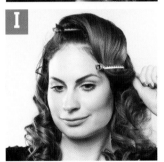

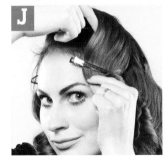

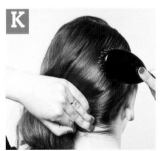

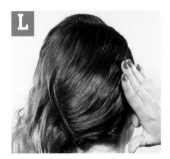

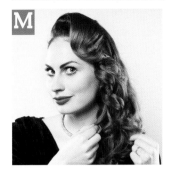

TIP

Alternative curling methods: A wet set roller would be perfect for creating defined curls, while small tongs or hot sticks would be a preferred heat method.

My hair is very fine: Add some extension wefts for length or volume. Pre-curl the wefts before you clip them to your head. Twist the roots and back-brush them gently before you clip in the extensions, providing a secure base for the brush-out. Remember the hair will be pulled to one side, so clip them to one side and put the comb further over to the smooth side to fit in the extensions.

I have a fringe: Curl the fringe section forwards into large pin curls in the same direction as the rest of the front section. The strong curl of the wet set should enable you to manipulate your fringe into the wave.

wave, smooth and make any adjustments to the shape. (J)

9. Once you are happy, grip into place.
10. Mist the front section with a firm-hold hairspray and leave to dry.
11. Sweep your hair to one side, smoothing with a bristle brush and add a large comb. (K,L)
12. Using your fingers, separate the hair into defined, sculpted curls. (M)
13. Finish the style with a mist of hairspray.

The Lamarr

This classic style with a centre parting was made popular by Hedy Lamarr and Vivien Leigh. It features smooth, defined waves with full body and curls at the bottom of the hair, and a smooth and sleek crown.

TECHNIQUES USED

Pin curls
Brushing into waves
Shaping with clips

KIT LIST

Pin curl clips
Setting lotion
Pomade
Hairspray
Styling brush
Tail comb
Kirby grips (optional)

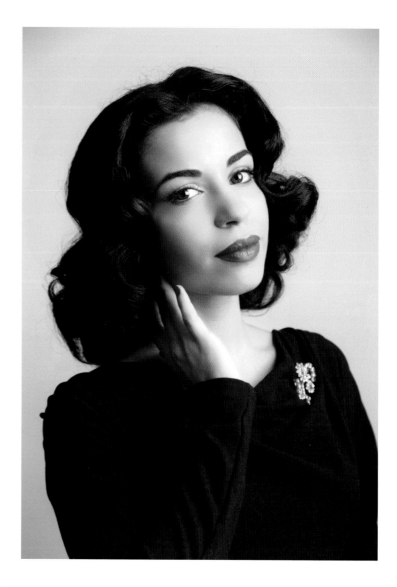

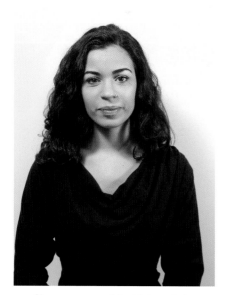

Shown on a model with long hair.

Directions

1. Set the hair in pin curls – see the specific pin curl pattern for this style. The crown is set in elevated pin curls rolling away from the face and in alternating rows at the back and sides. (A)
2. Remove the clips and separate the curls with your fingertips and some pomade. (B,C)
3. Brush the hair into waves, brushing the body of the curl to the ends of the hair. (D,E)
4. To keep the lift at the front of the hair, use your finger to support the hair whilst you brush it over and around your finger to shape the waves below. (F)
5. Continue brushing out the waves, using your fingers and duck-billed clips to shape them as you go. (G,H)
6. Once the waves are brushed through, use a tail comb to add more lift to the front section. (I)
7. Secure and shape the front with duck-billed clips. (J)
8. Mist with hairspray.
9. Remove the clips once the hairspray has dried.

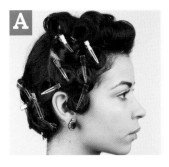

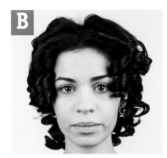

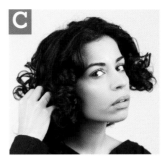

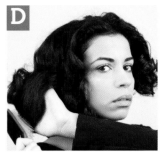

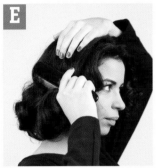

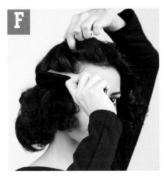

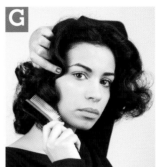

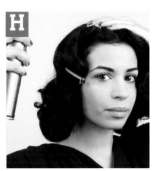

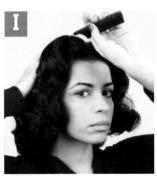

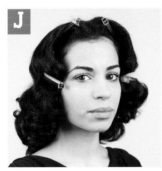

TIP

Alternative curling methods: Use medium Velcro or sponge rollers. Hot sticks or a small tong are the best heat option, but only use rollers if your hair responds very well to heat.

A centre parting doesn't suit me: This style can still work with an off-centre parting with the same setting pattern.

My hair is very fine: Add some extension wefts to create body and any desired length, setting the extensions with pin curls or Velcro rollers. Back-brushing can be used to add volume to the front and crown sections.

The Pageboy

This popular 1940s style continued to be worn by ladies well into the 1950s. All of the hair is curled towards the face and brushed under to create a smooth, sleek look. This style is best reproduced with pin curls, as they can be manipulated easily into the desired shape whilst providing the best holding power. It works well on various hair lengths, including shorter hair, providing there is sufficient length to roll over on itself once.

TECHNIQUES REQUIRED

Pin curls
Brushing in to waves
Unified wave

KIT LIST

Pin curl clips
Kirby grips
Hair comb
Hairspray
Pomade
Setting lotion
Styling brush
Hair net (optional)

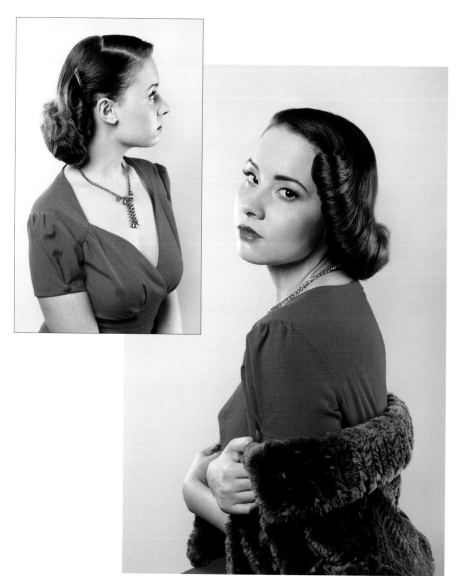

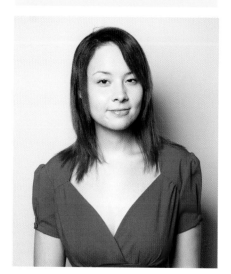

Shown on a model with medium-length hair.

Directions

1. Set the hair in small pin curls. Follow the pin curl diagram for this style. (A)
2. Separate the curls using your fingertips and some pomade. (B)
3. Start brushing through the curls with a styling brush, smoothing the hair onto your hand and tucking it underneath as you work around the head. (C,D,E)
4. Keep brushing, smoothing the hair at the front towards the face. (F)
5. After brushing through the back section and you can see the frizz is smoothing out, gather all the hair and hold firmly in one hand. Brush it together and use the unified wave technique to blend it in to one. (G,H)
6. Using your fingertips, gently spread the back section. (I,J)
7. Repeat this process until a smooth finish is achieved, with all the hair

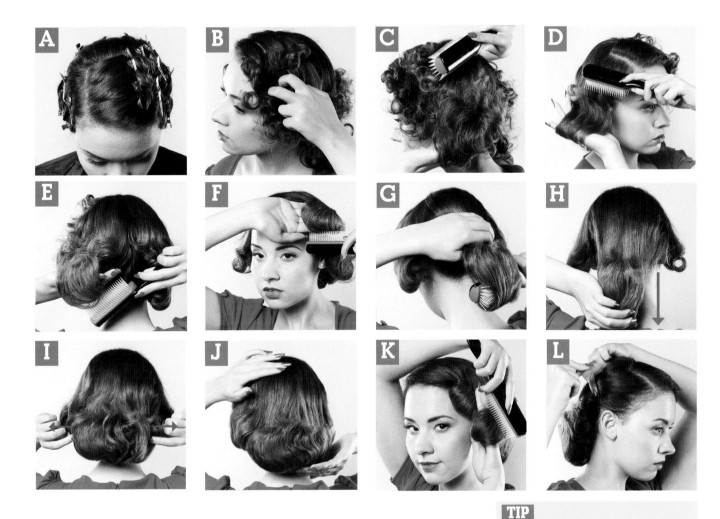

tucked under in a smooth wave.

8. Apply pomade to smooth the crown area and any flyaway hairs. Focus again on the front section, brushing both sides under and towards your face until soft barrel curls are formed. Make sure the front sections join the back by gently brushing them under together. (K)

9. Pull back the hair on the right side of the head and secure it with a comb. (L)

The Perfect Pomp

This look is based around the high pompadours and rolls style worn by Betty Grable. It is a style that you could wear day or evening, with smooth rolls contrasted by fluffy curls at the back. The front is pre-curled to give the style the height and volume it needs to create the pomp. To recreate this look you will need some hair length to create the large rolls at the front.

TECHNIQUES REQUIRED

Pin curls
Barrel Rolls
Victory Rolls
Fluff curls
Blending with hairpins

KIT LIST

Pomade
Hairspray
Hairpins
Kirby grips
Pin curl clips
Setting lotion
Styling brush
Bristle brush

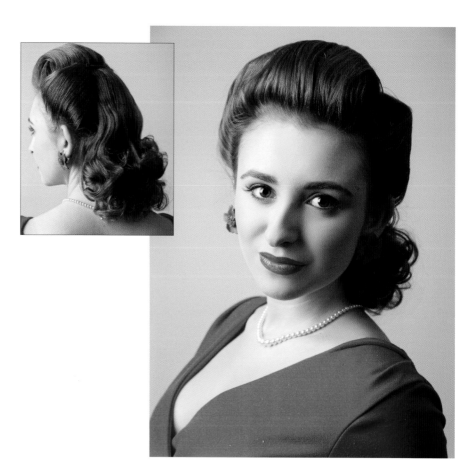

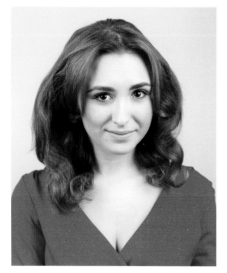

Shown on a model with medium-length hair.

Directions

1. Set the hair in pin curls, following the specific pattern for this style. The elevated pin curls all roll away from the face with the pin curls at the back all set in counter-clockwise curls. (A)
2. Remove the clips and separate through the curls with your fingertips and some pomade. Brush the back into fluff curls and smooth the crown section. (B,C,D)
3. Divide the front into three sections, parting the hair straight above the arch of each brow. Take the centre section and thoroughly back-brush it, one horizontal section at a time, giving it lots of volume. (E)
4. Lay the hair of the centre section over your hand. Make sure that you position your hand so it is directly

TIP

My hair isn't very long: Take a thinner section when you make the ear-to-ear parting. This means the roll will not have to be as wide to cover the parting.

My hair is very thick: Try making a smaller ear-to-ear parting so you are not overwhelmed with the amount of hair you have to work with.

My hair is very fine: Take an extra large section ear to ear. This will give you more hair to bulk out the pomp. Clip in wefts of extensions to add volume and/or length to the back. Try using some stuffing in the middle of the rolls to bulk them out.

I cannot cover the parting: Cover any flashes of parting with a couple or even a row of flowers behind the pomp.

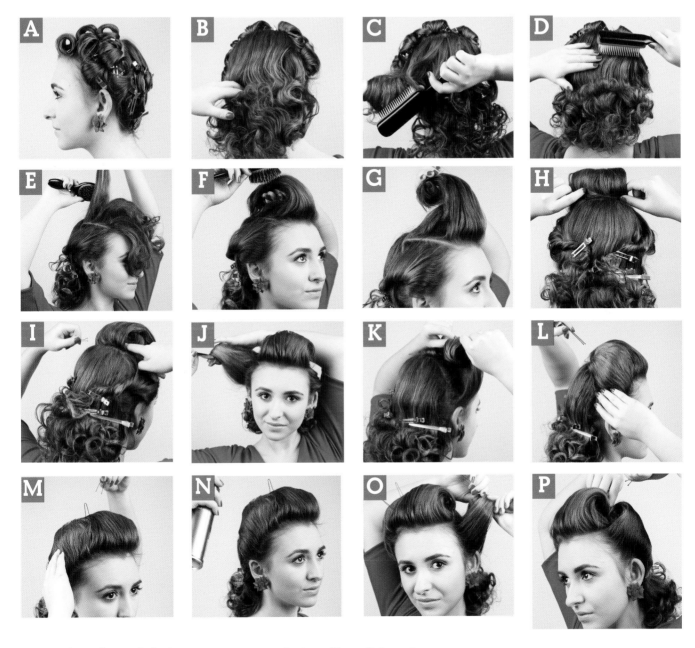

over the section, not far back or forward. Gently smooth the top layer. (F)

5. Roll the section into a large Barrel Roll, spreading the newly formed tube of hair with your fingertips, ensuring it covers the parting on the crown. (G,H)

6. Secure in place with grips. (I)

7. Back-brush the right hand side and roll it in to a Victory Roll, meeting the roll in the centre. (J,K)

8. Secure with grips and pins. (L)

9. Blend any gaps between the rolls with hairpins. (M,N)

10. Create a Victory Roll on the other side of the head and grip in to place. (O,P)

11. Use hairspray to set the hair and smooth any stray hairs.

The Pompadour Wave

This style is a variation of the Perfect Pomp, with the feature of a beautiful wave resting on the pompadour. The back is pulled up loosely into soft curls. The hair will need length to be pulled forward into the wave.

TECHNIQUES REQUIRED

Pin curls
Barrel Rolls
Victory Rolls
Fluff curls
Blending with pins

KIT LIST

Pomade
Hairspray
Hairpins
Kirby grips
Pin curl clips
Duck-billed clips
Styling brush
Setting lotion
Bristle brush

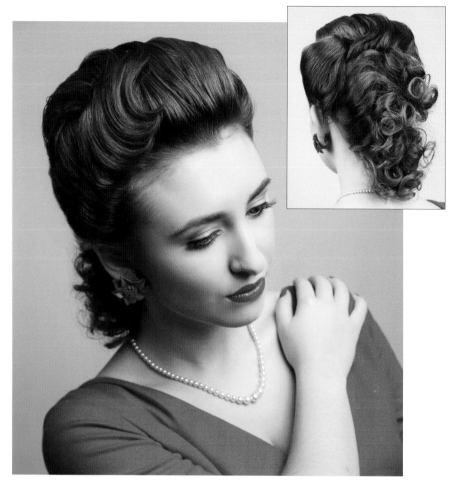

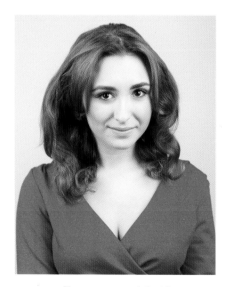

Shown on a model with medium-length hair.

Directions

1. Set the hair in pin curls, following the pin curl pattern for this style (*see* Appendix). The back of the head is set in counter-clockwise pin curls. The top of the head is set in four rows of elevated pin curls. The top three rows roll away from the face while the single back row rolls towards the face. (A)

2. Once the set has dried completely, clip the back row of elevated pin curls out of the way; you will dress it out later.

3. Next follow steps 2–10 from The Perfect Pomp tutorial. (B)

4. Once this is completed, unclip the back row of elevated pin curls remaining. Brush through the section thoroughly, brushing it on to your hand, working to remove and frizz. (C)

5. Hold the tip of the hair securely. Release the tension on the hair and you will see it fall naturally into a wave. (D)

6. Lay the wave on the pomp and use your fingertips to spread the wave. (E)

7. Use duck-billed clips to secure and accentuate the waves. Mist with hair spray. (F,G)

8. At the back, loosely pull up the side sections to create soft, cascading fluff curls. (H)

9. Smooth any stray hair and finish the style with a mist of hairspray.

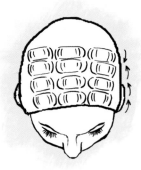

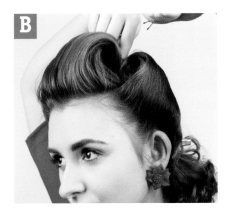

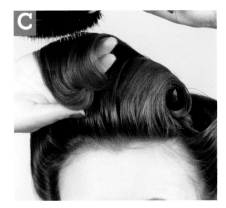

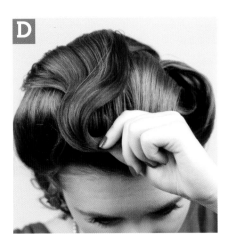

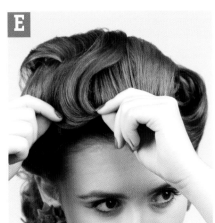

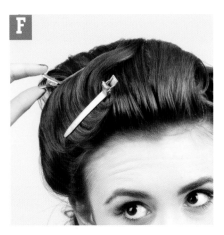

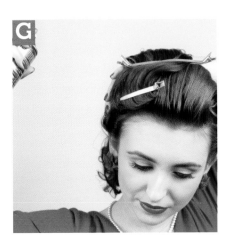

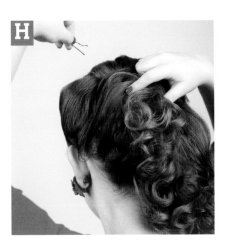

TIP

My hair isn't very long: Take thinner sections when you make the ear-to-ear parting. This means the roll will not have to be as wide to cover the parting.

My hair is very thick: Try making a smaller ear-to-ear parting so you are not overwhelmed with the amount of hair you have to work with.

My hair is very fine: Take an extra-large section ear to ear. This will give you more hair to bulk out the pomp. Clip in wefts or extensions to add volume and/or length to the back. Try using some stuffing in the middle of the rolls to bulk them out.

My hair won't spring in to the wave: Try using a smaller pin curl so you get a tighter curl.

The Bombshell

This classic style combines beautiful, soft curls with wide, structured waves. This look works perfectly for day and night and can be adapted for both long and very short hair.

The wet set allows you to manipulate and mould the hair into the defined waves with more ease than a hot set, without having to worry about the hair losing its curl.

TECHNIQUES USED

Pin curls
Elevated pin curls
Brushing into waves

KIT LIST

Pin curl clips
Duck-billed clips
Hairspray
Setting lotion
Pomade
Tail comb
Styling brush

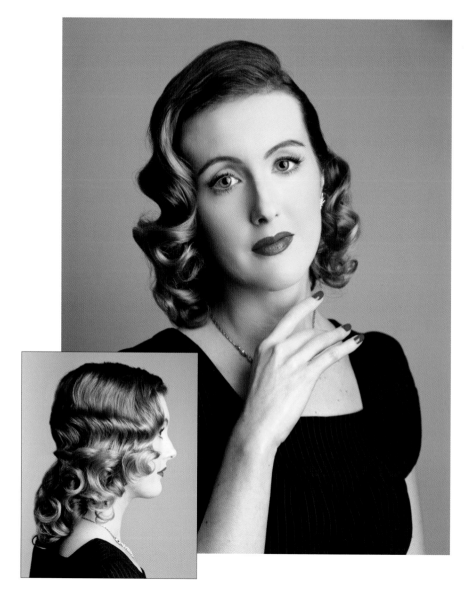

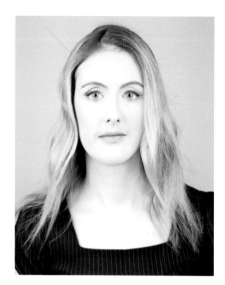

Shown on a model with long hair.

Directions

1. Set the hair in pin curls. Follow the specific setting pattern for this style with all of the pin curls set in alternating rows and the top in elevated pin curls. (A)
2. Separate the curls using your fingertips and some pomade. (B,C)
3. Brush the hair at the back and sides into soft curls and waves. (D,E)
4. A wave will start to form at the front; hold this in place with a duck-billed clip. (F)
5. Remove the pin curl clips from the front top section and separate the curls with your fingertips and some pomade. (G)
6. Lay the whole section over your hand and brush the hair together into waves. (H,I)
7. Use your fingertips to spread the waves widthways. (J)
8. Lay the side of your hand or a finger at the tip of each wave and, applying gentle pressure to the hair, move your hand towards and away

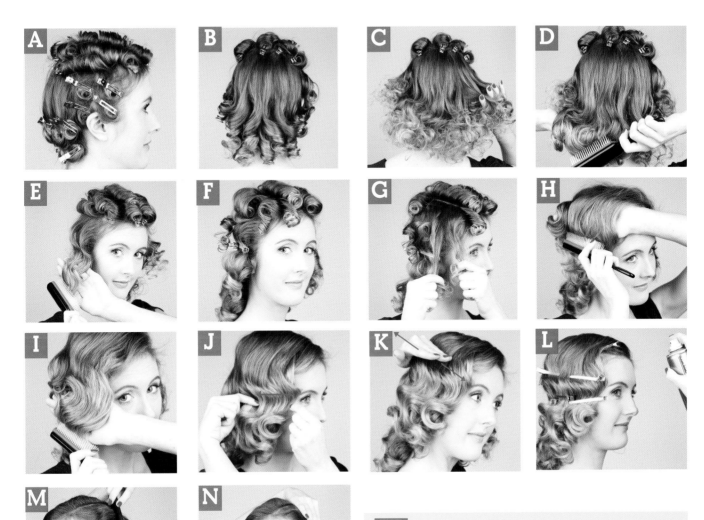

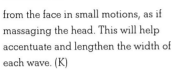

from the face in small motions, as if massaging the head. This will help accentuate and lengthen the width of each wave. (K)

9. Further define the waves by securing them with duck-billed clips and mist with hairspray. (L)

10. Comb the hair on the opposite side of the head away from the face, using spray to hold it in place. If you have thick hair, you may need to pin it into position. (M,N)

Glamour Girl

This smooth, sleek style features the details of a side wave flowing into a soft curl. Use a comb to accentuate and hold the ridges in place. The top section is given height and brushed into a smooth pompadour. The model has a side fringe, but this style could be recreated with or without one.

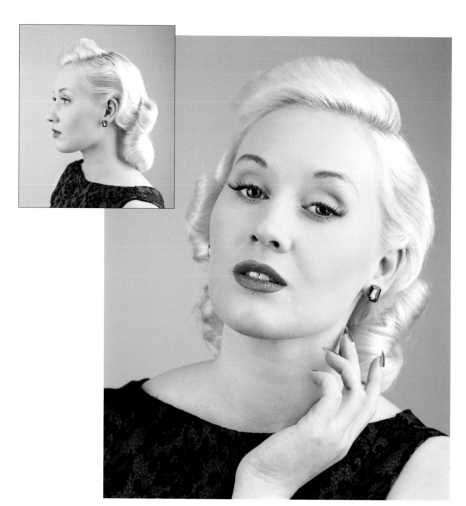

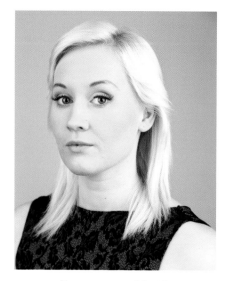

Shown on a model with medium-length hair.

Directions

1. Comb a ridge wave onto the side of the head, clipping in place to set and follow the pin curl pattern for this style. Form the ends of the ridge wave into medium pin curls that roll towards the face. The rest of the hair is set in medium pin curls rolling towards the face, while the crown is set in elevated pin curls all rolling backwards. (A)

2. Once the set is completely dry, remove the clips and separate the curls using your fingertips and some pomade. (B)

3. Brush through the hair with a styling brush. (C)

4. Brush through the wave. (D)

5. Use your hands to push the ridges of the wave back into shape after brushing through. (E,F)

6. Secure the wave with a duck-billed clip and hold securely as you brush out the curls below. (G,H)

7. Smooth all of the hair together and under into a sleek wave, using the unified wave technique. (I)

8. Brush the hair at the sides towards the face, forming sleek barrel curls. (J)

9. Smooth the top section into a soft pompadour. If you have fine hair, you may need to add some back-brushing to the base of the pompadour.

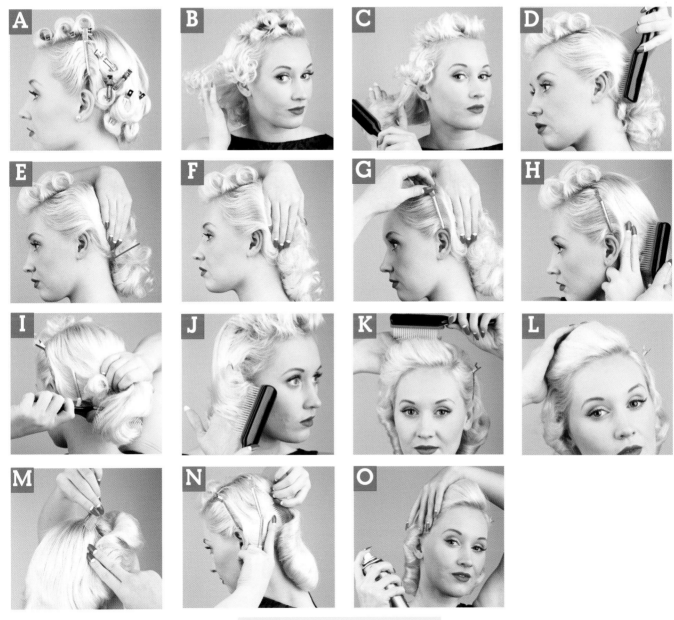

10. Secure the hair with a comb or grips. (K,L,M)

11. Repeat the process on the other side; the comb will hold the wave in place securely. (N)

12. Apply a mist of hairspray to complete the style. Once this is dry, remove the duck-billed clips. (O)

TIP

Alternative curling methods: Sponge or Velcro rollers are the best choice for a wet set. If using heat, hot sticks and tongs are a good method, or rollers if your hair responds well to heat.

My hair is very thick: Use a comb with a wider ridge to add in the waves. A duck-billed clip with teeth will hold the waves more firmly.

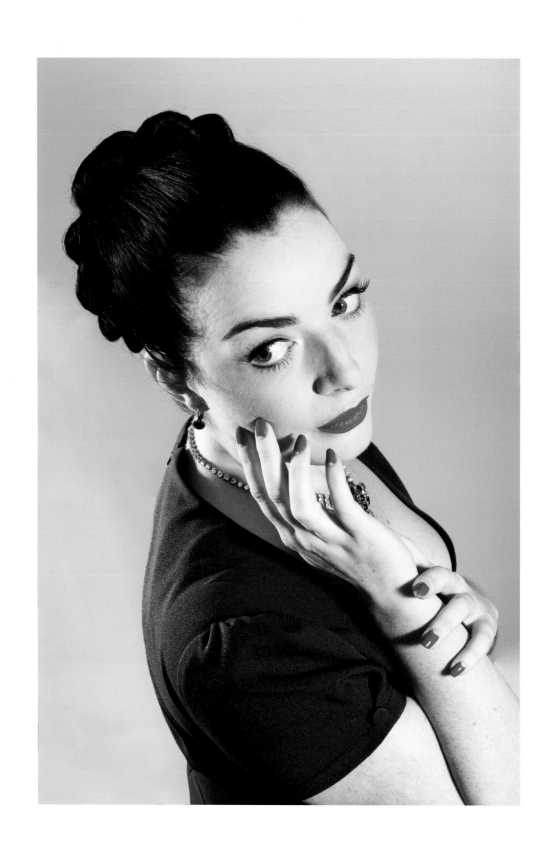

Chapter 8
Completing the Look

Hair Accessories

How to Tie a Head Scarf

Directions

1. Take a large, square headscarf and fold to create a triangle. Alternatively, choose a fabric you like, cut it to size and hem the edges.
2. Let the central triangular edge sit on your forehead, holding the two other edges out from the sides of your head. (A)
3. Pull the whole scarf downwards until you feel the straight edge sitting neatly at the bottom of your hairline. (B)
4. Tie the other two ends of the scarf securely up and over the front triangular point. (C)
5. Tuck the loose ends and any stray fabric into the pocket created on either side of the scarf. (D,E)
6. Tuck the triangular corner under the knot at the front of your head. (F)

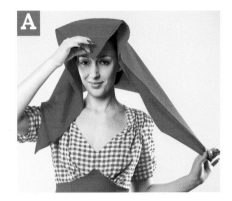

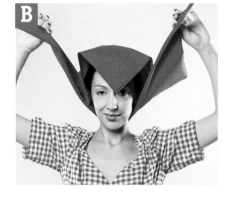

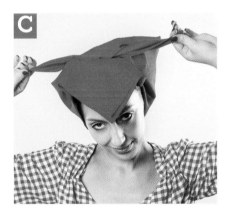

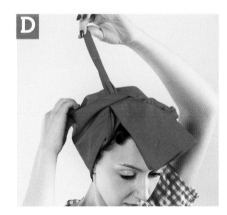

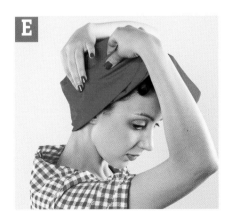

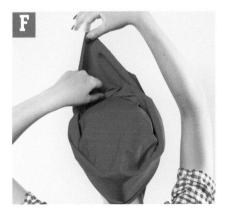

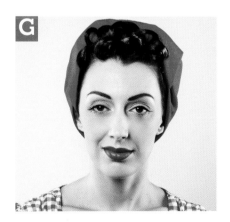

How To Tie a Turban

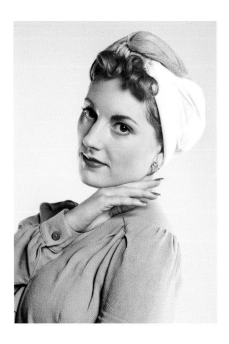

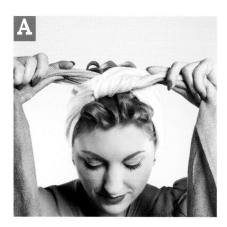

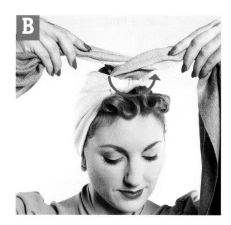

Directions

1. Take the piece of fabric or scarf and tie in a single knot on the crown of the head. (A)
2. Twist the ends anti-clockwise once around each other. (B)
3. Tuck the end on the right side of the head under the edge of the scarf. (C,D)
4. Tuck the other end over the top of the scarf on the opposite side of the head. (E,F)

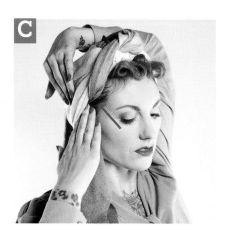

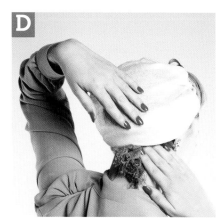

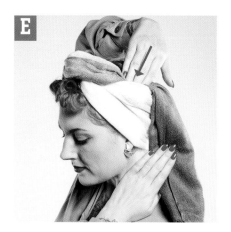

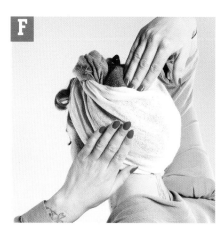

How To Make a Braided Hairpiece: Rope Braid

Purchase a packet of synthetic braid hair or 'pony braid' hair, or use real hair if you prefer. An elastic loop is used to secure the hair with grips, but you could skip this stage and pin into the braid if you wish.

A ribbon is used to decorate the plait, but you could experiment with pearls, scarves, flowers or even autumn leaves. This technique could be used to create other types of plaits, such as three- or four-strand braids.

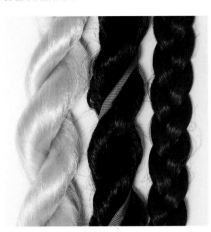

KIT LIST

Packet of synthetic hair

Small, clear elastic bands

Fabric, wide elastic or bias binding (in a corresponding colour)

Hot glue gun

Strong elastic hair bands

Directions

1. With the hair in one section, choose the thickness of your braid.
2. Wrap a few clear hair bands around all the hair strands at one end. Ensure the end is secured tightly. (A)
3. Get someone to hold the end for you or tie it temporarily to a secure surface. Divide the hair into two even sections. (B)
4. Twist both sections of hair separately

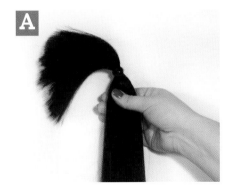

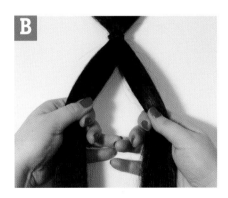

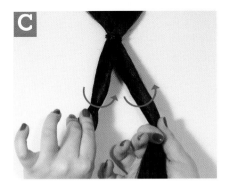

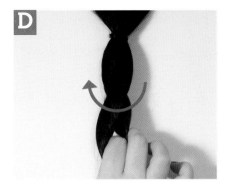

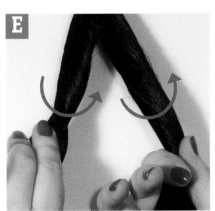

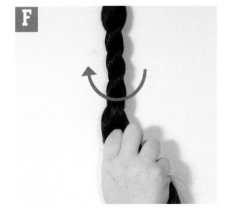

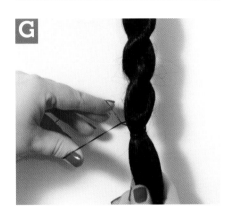

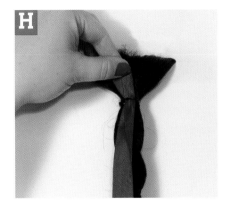

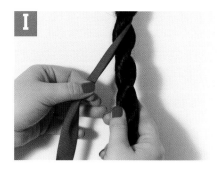

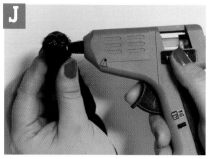

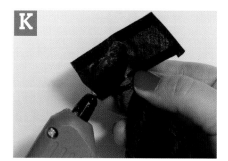

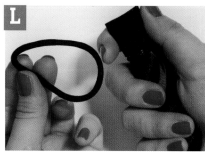

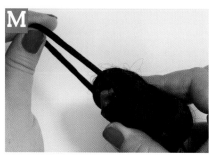

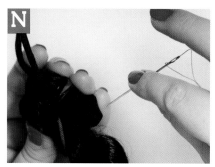

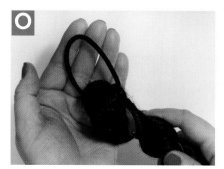

to the right. (C)

5. Next, twist the sections together as one; twisting both to the left. (D)

6. Repeat the twisting of both sections separately to the right and then twist both as one to the left. (E,F)

7. Repeat the process until you achieve the desired braid length. Secure the other end tightly with clear bands. (G)

8. If you wish to use ribbons or pearls to decorate the braid, simply tuck them under the elastic at one end and wrap around the braid, tucking the end under the band at the opposite end. The ribbon will naturally skip one dip in the braid as it is wrapped around. If you wish to use flowers you can stitch them on to the braid. (H,I)

9. Cut off the excess hair from each end with sharp scissors as neatly as possible, leaving around 1cm (0.5in) length from the band. Using a hot glue gun, cover the ends in glue to melt the ends of the synthetic hair. (J)

10. Using a piece of wide elastic, fabric or bias binding in a similar colour to the hair, use the glue gun and fabric to seal in the ends in a pocket. (K)

11. Take the strong hair band in a matching colour and fold the braid over it, leaving a small loop. (L,M)

12. With a thick needle and thread, stitch the fabric-covered end to the back of the braid, firmly securing the loop. (N)

13. Repeat the process on the other end. (O)

How to Make a Hair Rat

If you decide to make stuffing from your own hair, the colour and texture will be the same, thus allowing it to blend well if a corner of the rat decides to peek out.

Directions

1. Take a large handful of hair and roll it between your palms and fingers until it forms a firm ball (if you are using extension wefts, back-brush them for volume).

2. Next, pull the hair outwards into an oval, sausage shape, and roll it again until it is firm.

3. Wrap the hair in an old stocking or hairnet, doubling the hairnet over.

4. Seal the ends of the rat with a few stitches.

1940s Make-Up

Wartime rationing impacted on the hair and beauty products and services available to women during the conflict and the years that followed. Ingredients for make-up were sparse, with a dwindling supply of fats, oils and glycerine. Even soap was rationed. As well as the actual product, the packaging also was affected, as all metals were being used for the war effort. Moreover, glass was too expensive, paper proved ineffective and plastic was difficult to obtain.

Consequently, women had to improvise. Cherry juice was used in place of rouge and as a lip stain. Alternatively, a solution of cooked beetroot topped with Vaseline made a good lipstick. Talcum powder and powdered starch replaced some specialist face powders and, in the absence of foundation, calamine lotion was mixed with cold cream to create a base for the powder. Burnt cork was used as mascara.

To overcome the shortage of stockings, leg make-up became an inexpensive and frequently used solution. This was known as liquid or bottle stockings and could be purchased from companies such as Max Factor and Elizabeth Arden; the latter boasted twenty pairs from each 5oz bottle. In the United States, some department stores even featured leg

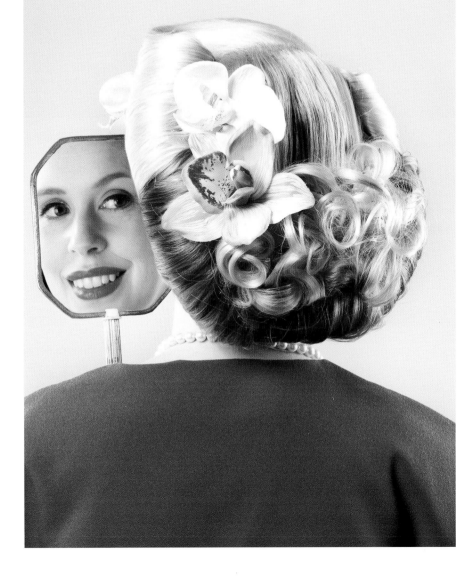

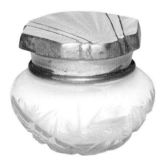

Cold cream.

make-up parlours or bars in which you could purchase a bottle of 'phantom hose' and get advice on the proper application. Many women improvised their own recipes, such as diluted gravy browning and using eye liner to add seams to the backs of their legs.

The advertising for Tangee, a vintage lipstick brand, featured a uniformed Wren alongside the strapline: 'For Beauty on Duty'. Similarly, British make-up brand Cyclax aimed their products at

the forces, introducing the provocatively named 'Auxiliary Red' lipstick and rouge in 1939. The tube was designed to fit perfectly in the uniform pockets of servicewomen. Some believe that this campaign started the trend for the bright red lipsticks commonly seen during the war.

The tip of the lipstick was known as 'the bullet' due to its resemblance to an ammunition round. This ingenious wartime marketing was bolstered by the

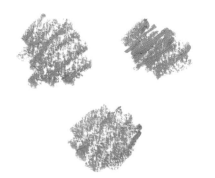

1940s lip colours.

fact that Cyclax also actively contributed to the war effort. The company developed a special lotion for the treatment of burns, a sun protection cream for soldiers fighting in hot climates and a camouflage cream for covering up wounds. It was during this time that certain make-up brands started to realize how popular camouflage products could be and these formed the basis for the concealers that would be used by women in the future.

Once the war was over and the initial lull in manufacturing ceased, make-up production began to increase again and by the end of the decade women had a whole new host of colours and products to play with.

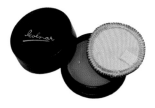

1940s rouge.

The Look

In contrast to the bee-stung pouts and fine arched eyebrows of the 1930s, the fashion for make-up in the 1940s was a softer, more natural and pared down look.

The 1940s glamour guide *Beauty*,

Glamor and Personality explains:

'the secret of successful make up is naturalness, the closest possible adherence to nature's own handiwork, the coloration and facial delineation intended by nature itself.'[11]

Excessive make-up was considered unfashionable and even frowned upon by some. Heavy eyeshadow and mascara, harsh rouge and lipstick:

'give the whole face an appearance of artificiality – a 'painted' look.'[12]

Eyebrows were pencilled lightly and importance was placed on following the natural contour of the brow, with a fuller look and long, sculpted arches. Emphasis was given to the lashes, which were long, defined and curled to open the eye. False lashes were natural and tapered at the edges to provide thickness and length. Eyeshadow, if used, was mostly in soft brown or grey shades, but it was a rarity for most and saved for evening wear. After the war, more colours of shadow were introduced, such as blues and greens, but application remained light and minimal.

The lower lash line was always free from liner, giving a clean and fresh look. Mascara was also sometimes skipped on the bottom lash. At times, the upper lash line had a very fine line of liner or powder, but this was kept minimal to avoid a 'painted' look and was more

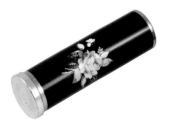

Decorative lipstick tube.

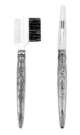

1940s make-up brushes.

prevalent in the late 1940s.

Lips were fuller, following a more natural lip line. The top lip was sometimes accentuated in a soft, heart shape, rounding out the Cupid's bow. This style was called the hunter's bow and was popularized by Joan Crawford's full and lavish pout. A lip brush was used to achieve a precise shape and reds in a variety of shades were the most popular colours. Ladies were told:

'lipstick is your exclamation point ... use it sparingly but well.'[13]

Red lipstick was regarded as a sign of patriotism during the 1940s and importance was placed on keeping up appearances during the war. Not only did a bright red lipstick make ladies feel more feminine, it also gave them the confidence to defy the difficult and austere times.

Popular rouge colours included pink, peach and coral, with the aim being to achieve a natural, rosy look. One beauty expert advised:

'If you wear rouge, try putting it on with the tridot system. One dot directly under the pupil of the eye, the second dot directly under the cheekbone and the third no lower than the tip of the nose. Now fill in the triangle lightly and blend until no-one can see that the rouge is there, not even you.'[14]

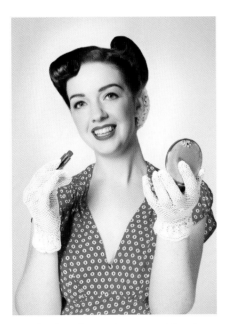

Bright red lipstick was considered 'patriotic'.

A matte finish on the skin was popular, especially with the new pancake make-up introduced by Max Factor. The advertising campaign was fronted by Rita Hayworth and promised the wearer would 'gain more loveliness and create the glamour you desire' with this 'gift from Hollywood'. A pressed powder compact or loose powder was used to set the foundation.

This following sections will provide instructions for creating an authentic 1940s look using modern products and

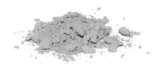

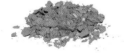

Popular rouge colours.

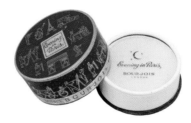

Vintage powder.

tools. We will break down the kit required to recreate a classic make-up look and what to consider when selecting products.

Tools

POWDER PUFF
Apply powder with a puff. Dip the puff into the powder then tap it on the back of your hand a couple of times to remove any excess powder. If you are using pressed powder, push the puff gently into the powder to load it.

Press and roll the puff onto your skin to apply the powder. Avoid making any rubbing or buffing motions as this will unsettle the foundation and concealer already applied. Use a powder brush to sweep away any excess powder from the surface of the skin.

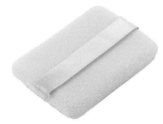

Vintage powder puff.

LIP BRUSH
Using a brush rather than the 'bullet' of the lipstick gives you more control to apply and shape your lips to perfection. A foldaway brush is perfect for touch-ups on the go.

FLAT-ANGLE BRUSH
This is used with powder, gel or wax for precise eyebrow application. Slowly build up the shape and depth of colour, taking care not to overload with product.

This brush is also available in fine widths, which can be used to apply liner to the upper lid. Push the brush into shadow or gel liner and then repeatedly press the brush onto the lash line, creating a soft line.

LINER BRUSH
Use this brush for the precise application of gel or liquid liner. If you have shaky hands, try resting your elbow on the dressing table as you work; this will help steady any wobbles. Have a pointed cotton bud and make-up remover on hand to quickly fix any mistakes before the liner dries.

BLENDING/FLUFF BRUSH
This soft brush has a round, moulded shape, which is perfect for blending shadow and removing harsh lines. Ensure the brush is clean and free of shadow before you start blending. The brush is also great at blending and buffing concealer around the eyes, ensuring the area is covered without overloading it with product.

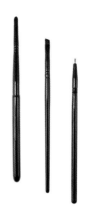

Left to right: lip brush, flat angle brush, liner brush.

PENCIL/CREASE BRUSH

A pencil brush is used for applying shadow to the crease before blending out with a blending brush. The pointed tip enables precise application.

CONCEALER BRUSH

This small, flat brush is perfect for precise concealer application under the eyes and on blemishes.

POWDER BRUSH

This brush can be used both to apply and remove excess powder. Be sure to use pressing motions, rather than rubbing, to avoid unsettling the foundation and concealer already applied.

CONTOUR BRUSH

This angled brush can be used in the place of a blusher brush. It is shaped to fit the contours of the face, which is good for shading and adding definition to the cheekbones. It can also be used to apply powder and for blending blusher.

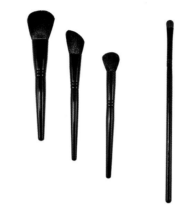

Left to right: powder brush, contour brush, blusher brush, flat eyeshadow brush.

BLUSHER BRUSH

This soft brush with a rounded tip can be used to buff blusher evenly onto the skin. Make gentle circular motions to blend the blusher evenly.

FLAT EYE SHADOW BRUSH

Use this brush to apply shadow directly to the lid and brow bone evenly.

FOUNDATION BRUSH

There are many different types, but the most popular are a flat foundation brush or stippling brush. The flat foundation brush is good for applying liquid or cream foundation. The tapered edge is useful when blending foundation into hard to reach areas, such as around the

eyes or hairline. The stippling brush is good for all types of foundation and is used in circular motions to buff the foundation into the skin, producing a flawless effect. This buffing motion also means you are left with no foundation streaks.

First, apply your foundation in a fine layer; then use concealer where it is needed. This produces a more natural, radiant look.

FALSE EYELASHES

Pick natural lashes that taper at the edges or glue a few individual lashes on the edges of your eyes for an authentic look.

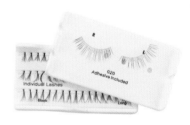

False eyelashes.

Eyelash Curlers

Use these to curl and define your lashes. Gently squeeze the lashes rather than clamp them, working your way up the lash.

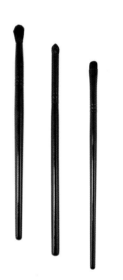

Left to right: fluff brush, pencil brush, concealer brush.

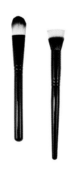

Flat foundation brush, stippling brush.

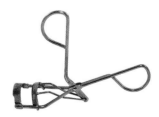

Eyelash curlers.

Products

PRIMERS
Primers help to secure make-up and provide a smooth base on which to apply the make-up. For the face, buy a primer suited to your needs, such as moisturizing, oil-free or pore-reducing. Eyelid primers stop the shadow from creasing and wearing away.

FOUNDATION
Choose a foundation to suit your skin type, bearing in mind that the fashion in the 1940s for skin was shine-free and matte. However, if you have dry skin, avoid purchasing a very matte foundation as it will be even more drying; buy a more moisturizing formula and ensure it is powdered well.

CONCEALER
Concealer is used to cover blemishes, redness and any other flaws on the skin. Always set the concealer by firmly pressing powder over the top.

POWDER
Use powder to set your foundation and concealer and remove shine during the day. If you have oily skin and you need to reapply often, a translucent powder avoids the skin appearing 'cakey' due to a build-up of coloured powder.

SETTING SPRAY
Setting spray is used at the end of the process to hold the make-up in place, especially in hot and humid environments. Many formulas contain alcohol, so avoid using every day if you have sensitive/dry skin and save for special occasions.

EYESHADOW
Pick a highly pigmented shadow as this will produce a better result with less need for as large amount of product. Use a matte shadow for an authentic look. A matte cream shadow could be used for dehydrated or dry skin.

BROW POWDER
Usually, these come in palettes with two shades so you can match your brows exactly by blending the colours. If you have wayward brows, fix them with a clear gel or wax. You can also use a matte eye shadow if you find a good match for your brows.

BLUSHER
A powder formulation is good for most, although, if you have dry skin, a cream or gel blusher is best.

EYELINER
Liners come in various guises, including gel, pen and liquid. Experiment and see which you prefer; the important factor is to choose something that allows you to create a thin, precise line.

LIPSTICK
In the 1940s lipstick had a matte finish. Picking lipstick with a matte or semi-matte finish will make your look last longer, as glossy formulas slide off easily. Adding a liner all over the lips before applying the lipstick will add longevity.

PICKING YOUR PERFECT RED
Blue red: Classic red with a cooler, blue base. Looks striking on pale and medium skin tones.

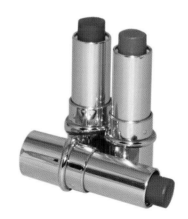

Left to right: blue red, coral red, true red.

Coral red: Coral red with hints of orange. Works on most skin tones but is perfect for medium and olive skin.
True red: Suits most skin tones. Compliments beautifully skin with a yellow tone, as well as dark and bronzed skin.

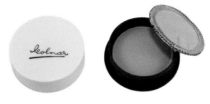

Peach blusher.

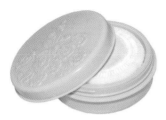

Vintage powder pot.

Creating the Look

Directions

1. Let your moisturizer absorb completely before applying foundation. Apply a base of foundation all over your face, keeping the application light and blending well. Using a primer first will help the foundation last.
2. Use a concealer to cover up any blemishes and dark circles under the eyes.
3. Set the foundation by pressing powder onto your face with a powder puff; then remove any excess powder by very gently dusting your face with a clean powder brush.
4. Dab an eyelid primer over the lid. Using a flat eyeshadow brush, sweep a neutral-coloured, matte shadow over the lid and brow-bone. (A)
5. With a pencil brush, apply a small amount of darker shadow to your natural crease. To find this, half close your eye and touch your eyeball; you will feel where your eye meets the bone of your eye socket. This is where you will place the darker shadow, following the line of your eye socket in a side-to-side motion. Place the shadow from the outer corner of your eye to two-thirds along your socket line, taking care to avoid the inner corner of your eye. (B,C)
6. Take a clean blending brush. Starting from the outer corner and working in, move the brush in tiny circles to gently blend the darker and lighter shadow. Next, blend in the other direction, sweeping back and forth in the crease of your eye. Continue these motions until you have blended all harsh lines. If you wish to create a more intense look, simply add more of the darker shadow to the crease with the pencil brush and repeat the blending

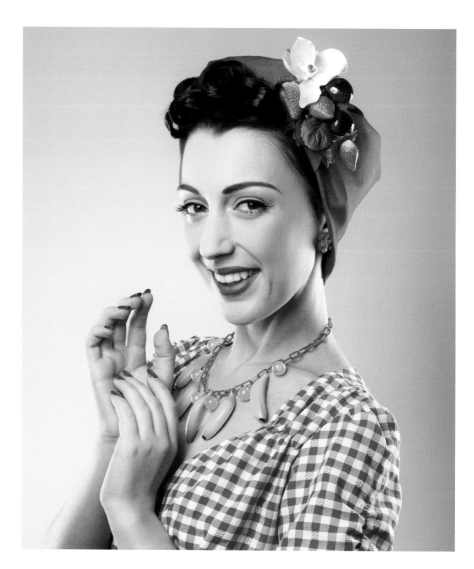

process until you are happy with the result. (D)

7. Line the top lash with a fine layer of gel liner or use a brown or black shadow with a flat-angle brush and push powder along the lash line. (E)
8. Curl your lashes and apply a layer of mascara.
9. Add individual lashes from the centre of the eye outwards. You could also use a natural-looking strip lash if you prefer. Blend the false lashes with your own using a thin coat of mascara. (F)
10. Using a flat-angle brush and brow powder, shape the brows into a long and sculpted arch. A pencil can be used if you prefer, but be careful to avoid an overly harsh look. (G)
11. Ensure the lip is totally free of balm or oil and line your lips with a sharp pencil. For extra longevity, cover the whole lip area with the pencil. (H)
12. Apply lipstick with a brush. After one coat, blot. Then apply another coat and blot again. (I)
13. Finish the look with a sweep of blusher, starting from the apples of the cheeks and blending upwards towards the ears. (J)

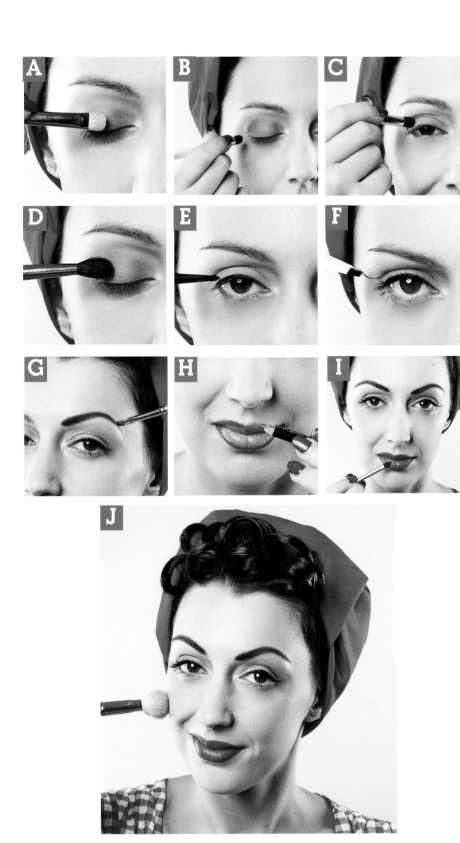

TIP

Do not: use too much product. Overloading on primer and shadow can create the appearance of 'cakey' lids. Use a quality, highly pigmented product so you do not have to add multiple layers of shadow.

Too much foundation makes the skin look cakey. Apply a fine layer and conceal where it is needed.

Applying a thick layer of lipstick in one go will make it slide off, so work a thin layer into the lip for a long-lasting look.

I have a wobbly lip line: Tidy and sharpen edges with a dab of concealer on a concealer brush.

I cannot get my liner straight/it is too thick: Steady a wobbly hand by resting your arm on the dressing table as you apply. Personally, I apply my liner with my eye open whilst looking in the mirror. This gives me control over the end result, as opposed to applying with your eye shut.

The concealer under my eyes goes into creases: Keep your application light, buffing the concealer into the skin. As soon as you have applied the concealer, take a puff loaded with a fine layer of powder (ensure you thoroughly knock off the excess) and, whilst looking upwards and holding a hand mirror, roll and press the powder with the puff onto the concealer under your eyes. Gently brush off any excess with a powder brush or clean fluff brush.

Too much blusher: If you have applied too much blusher or have obvious lines, take a clean blusher or contour brush and gently buff the edges of the blusher, blending it softly. Buffing over the blusher with powder will also tone it down.

1940s Nails

Ladies in the 1940s took care of their nails. Just as effort was placed in maintaining a hairstyle, nails were kept neat and well manicured. The fashion was to file the fingernail tip into an oval or 'almond' shape.

In terms of colours, 'crème' finishes, the glossy-looking nail polishes of one uniform colour, were most prevalent and are those you would use to recreate an authentic look. While reds, pinks and neutral shades were popular, a whole host of other colours were worn from yellows through to blacks. An advert for 'Chen U Nails' in 1945 showcased new unusual colours such as: 'Blue Dragon', 'Green Dragon', 'Ming Yellow' and 'Black Lustre'.

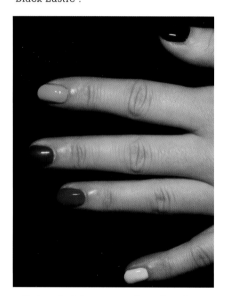

Red and pink were not the only colour choices for nails.

Long nails were often painted in one solid colour, but fine-detail nail art also saw a rise to prominence throughout this period. In the US, 'patriotic manicures' were advertised in women's magazines with nail decals/transfers of flags, Jeeps, initials and other designs becoming available.

Extremely popular was the 'half moon

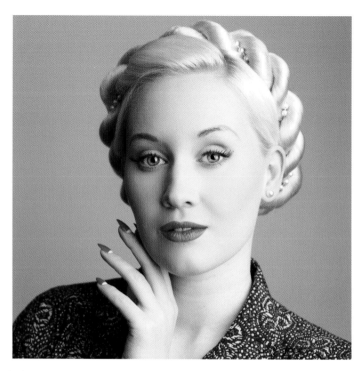

manicure' in which the crescent-shaped area at the base of the nail, known as the lanula, was left bare and the rest of the nail painted in a chosen colour. Sometimes a sliver of nail was also left bare at the tip.

HALF MOON MANICURE
Directions
1. File your nails into an oval/almond shape.
2. Push your cuticles back with a cuticle pusher. You can do this dry or with a cuticle remover. If you do not have a cuticle pusher, just wrap an orange stick in some cotton wool and gently push back. (A)
3. Wash your hands, dry them and paint on your chosen base coat. (B)
4. Use a fine nail art brush to create the moon shape at the top of the nail. (C)
5. Fill in the rest of the nail with downward strokes. (D)
6. Brush on a top coat and leave to dry thoroughly. (E)
7. Finish with some cuticle oil. (F)

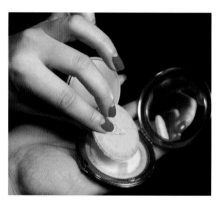

Classic half moon manicure.

TIP **THE HALF MOON CHEAT TECHNIQUE**

If you are finding difficulty with drawing the half moon freehand, then you can try using a guide. You can buy guides that are used for French manicures, but I find the best and most thrifty choice for a guide are the paper hole re-enforcers that you get from stationery shops as these are the perfect shape.

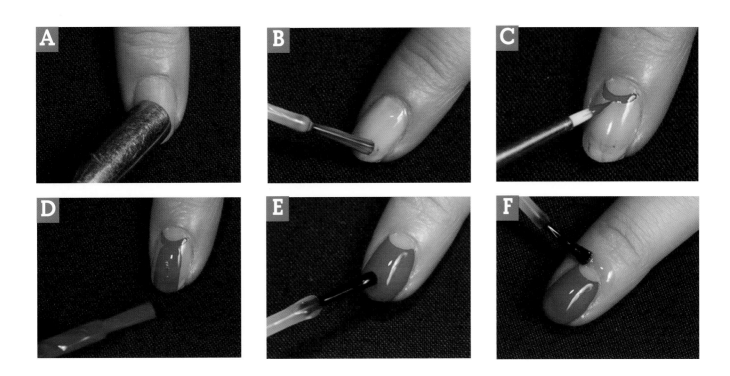

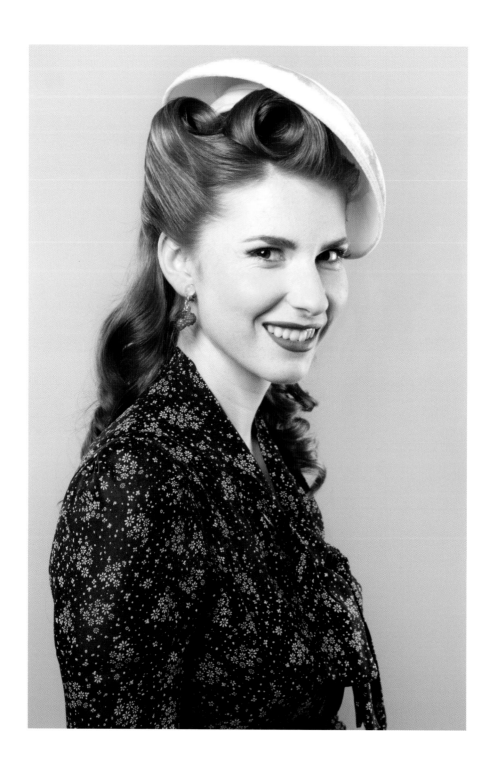

Chapter 9
Home-made Lotions and Potions

*Before reaching for shop-bought products,
which are often full of chemicals,
experiment with creating your own
simple, effective and affordable hair and
beauty treatments.*

*The recipes below have been used,
adapted and passed down through the
generations. Ancient Greeks used similar
recipes by seeping herbs and flowers in
vinegar and oil, or mixing them with
beeswax to create pomades for the face
and body, while my Grandma swore by her
vinegar hair rinse and how it made her
silvery locks shine.*

*All the ingredients used in these recipes
were available to ladies in the 1940s,
although some were harder to obtain or
used specifically for consumption due to
wartime shortages and rationing.*

Setting Lotions

Beer Setting Lotion

Beer is a great setting lotion. The
proteins in the malt and hops nourish
and repair damaged hair while
providing a volume boost.
Simultaneously, the sugars in the beer
tighten the cuticles in the hair shaft,
giving a beautiful shine

Leave the beer to go flat overnight (a
light beer is best). Put a small amount in
a spray bottle and mist lightly over each
section of hair before rolling. The aroma
will dissipate as the beer dries.

Allow the set to dry fully, preferably
overnight. Brush out into fluffy, shiny
curls.

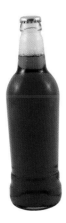

Sugar Water Setting Lotion

Dissolve 2tsp of sugar in 125ml of water.
Add to a spray bottle and mist over the
hair before pin-curling or rolling with
rags or rollers. Allow the set to dry fully
before brushing out, preferably
overnight.

Linseed Setting Lotion

Linseeds are packed full of essential fatty
acids that leave the hair nourished, soft
and shiny. This simple setting lotion
gives the hair great hold with no
crunchiness, flaking or drying effects.

Ingredients:
1tbsp linseed (also known as flax
seeds)
250ml water
A couple of drops of essential oil
(optional)
A couple of drops of vitamin E
(optional)

Directions
1. Place the flax seeds and water in a
   small pan and mix. Bring the
   mixture to a boil. Simmer for 10
   minutes until the mixture thickens

A WORD OF CAUTION:

- Skin-test all recipes before use on your
  jawline or inner arm to test for any skin
  sensitivities.
- Keep all remedies and treatments out of
  the eyes.
- If irritation occurs, stop treatment
  immediately.
- All recipes are obtained and adapted
  from historical sources or word of
  mouth.

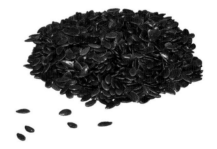

and become gelatinous. Take the
mixture off the heat and strain
immediately, discarding the seeds.
Add a couple of drops of essential
oil if you wish to add a scent to the
setting lotion; I like rose or orange.
2. Leave the mixture to cool – it will be
   the texture of egg whites. Store the
   mixture in the fridge where it will
   last a few days. A drop of vitamin E
   oil will help prolong its shelf life. If
   you have an excess or you want to
   make a large batch, store the
   prepared setting lotion in the freezer
   in ice cube trays and take it out as

3. Apply to damp hair (do not apply to very wet hair or it will never dry). If you hair is thick and you know it takes a long time to dry fully, try applying the mixture to dry hair.

4. Divide the hair into your usual sections for setting. Using your fingers, apply a small amount of the mixture to each section, then comb through the hair to remove any excess lotion. You do not want to overload the hair with the gel. Pin curl, rag or roll as normal. As with any wet set, ensure the hair is completely dry before brushing out.

Hair Treatments

Egg Masks

Eggs do wonders for the hair. The yolk, rich in fat and protein, is a natural moisturizer and nourishes dry, damaged hair, while the egg white, containing bacteria-eating enzymes, works to remove unwanted oils. Vitamins A and E contribute to preventing hair-thinning and hair loss, while Vitamin D helps to improve the hair's texture, shine and health. In addition the sulphur present in the yolks can help in the treatment of dandruff.

Eggs were rationed in June 1941, so were difficult to obtain during the war years, although they were easier to obtain in rural areas.

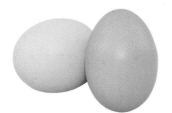

NORMAL HAIR
Whisk one egg, or two if you have long hair. Apply to the hair, paying special attention to the lengths and ends. Wrap your hair in a towel and leave for 30 minutes. Rinse thoroughly with lukewarm/cool water (using hot water runs the risk of cooking the yolk on your head!)

DRY HAIR
Whisk 1–4 egg yolks together depending on the thickness and length of your hair. Wrap your hair in a towel and leave for 30 minutes. Rinse thoroughly with lukewarm/cool water.

OILY HAIR
Whisk 1–3 egg whites together, depending on the thickness and length of your hair. Wrap your hair in a towel and leave for 30 minutes. Rinse thoroughly with lukewarm/cool water.

Honey Masks

Honey is extremely nourishing as it is a humectant and emollient, which means it helps to retain moisture in the hair whilst softening and smoothing. As a result, it is a great conditioner. Honey also has antibacterial and antioxidant properties, and is full of nutrients; therefore, it is beneficial to scalp health and promoting hair growth.

Raw honey is unheated, unpasteurized and unprocessed. Choose this over processed honey as all the vitamins, enzymes and nutrients are preserved.

BASIC HONEY MASK
Ingredients:
2tbsp honey
Water (optional)

Directions
Apply the honey to the hair and scalp, and massage thoroughly. If the honey is very solid, add a dash of warm water to

loosen it and make it easier to apply. Wrap the hair in a hot towel or cover with a shower cap. Leave to work in the hair for around an hour. Wash hair as normal.

MILK AND HONEY HAIR MASK
Milk is high in protein and perfect for nourishing brittle, damaged, thin hair that is easily weighed down by conditioners and oil treatments. However, it also has benefits for all hair types.

Ingredients:
400ml whole milk
2tsp honey

Directions
Gently warm the milk; do not boil or get it scalding hot. Add the honey and stir until it is dissolved. Pour the solution over dry hair, massaging from root to tip to ensure full coverage. If you have long hair, dip the ends of your hair in a jug containing the mixture before pouring over the rest of your hair. Cover your hair with a shower cap and leave for 15–30 minutes. Wash hair as normal.

HONEY MASK FOR DRY OR CURLY HAIR
In the 1940s olive oil was available for purchase only in pharmacies. The oil contains fatty acids that will coat the shaft of your hair, giving it a sleeker, smoother and healthier appearance, and helping repair any heat or chemical damage.

Ingredients:
2tbsp honey
2tbsp olive oil

Directions
Mix the honey and olive oil together. Apply to dry hair, massaging from root to tip. Cover your head with a very warm towel for 30 minutes, or longer for

very damaged hair. Shampoo the hair as normal.

Hot Oil Treatments

Hot oil treatments are great for use on all hair types and a weekly hot oil treatment will help keep your hair silky and smooth. Hot oil treatments can be done with oil alone or you can tailor your own hot oil blend by creating a herbal infusion for your hair type.

FOR OILY HAIR
Use castor oil mixed with a few drops of lemon juice.

FOR NORMAL HAIR
Use castor oil.

FOR DRY HAIR
Use olive oil.

STIMULATING SCALP AND HAIR HOT OIL TREATMENT
Rosemary and lavender are high in antioxidants and both have great antibacterial properties. Their use on the scalp helps to clean the hair follicles and stimulate healthy growth.

Mint is ideal for stimulating circulation to the hair follicles and provides an energy boost to the hair and scalp. Furthermore, it helps to control excessive oil production, so is perfect for use on oily hair.

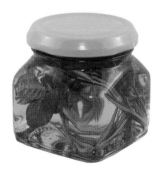

Ingredients:
Castor oil or oil of your choice
Rosemary (1–2 sprigs)
Mint (1–2 sprigs)
Lavender (1–2 sprigs)

Directions
Sterilize a small jar by filling it with boiling water and leaving to air dry. Place 1–2 sprigs of each herb in the jar. A teaspoon of each dried herb can be used as an alternative to fresh. Cover the herbs with your castor oil and leave to set for 2–3 weeks, shaking the contents from time to time to encourage the herbs to infuse. Strain the mixture before using.

MOISTURIZING HOT OIL TREATMENT
Chamomile has great healing, antioxidant and moisturizing properties, so it works wonders on dehydrated hair and scalps in need of some nourishment.

Ingredients:
Olive oil
2 tablespoons chamomile leaves or 4 chamomile tea bags

Directions
Sterilize a small jar by filling it with boiling water and leaving to air dry. Place the chamomile in the jar. Cover the herbs with olive oil and leave to set for 2–3 weeks, shaking the contents from time to time to encourage the herbs to infuse. Strain the mixture before using.

APPLYING HOT OILS
1. Warm the oil by placing it in a jar of very hot water. Leave for 2 minutes and carefully remove.
2. Starting at the scalp, apply the oil to your hair and massage in order to stimulate circulation and help absorb the oil. (Test a dab of the oil on your wrist first to check that it is not too hot.) Continue applying the oil to the lengths of your hair, taking

care not to overload the hair with oil. A small amount will be sufficient.
3. Cover your hair with a shower cap and wrap in a warmed towel (you can warm the towel by running it under hot water and wringing it out thoroughly). Once it has cooled, replace it with a dry towel.
4. Leave the solution to work its magic for 25 minutes to 3 hours. In extreme cases of very dry and damaged hair, leave the oil to work overnight.
5. Rinse thoroughly with shampoo – two rinses may be necessary if you can still feel the oil on your hair. Once you have rinsed out the shampoo, give your hair a final rinse with cool water.
6. If your hair is long, clip it up out of the way and wash the excess oil off your neck and back to ensure it does not transfer to your clean hair. If your hair feels dry (though most likely it will not), condition as normal.

Hair Rinses

CIDER VINEGAR HAIR RINSE

Vinegar removes product residue and scaly build-up from the hair shaft, closing the cuticles. Excess residue and open hair shafts render hair dull and lifeless, while a smoother cuticle yields shiny and healthy hair with fewer tangles. Vinegar also stimulates circulation to the scalp, which promotes

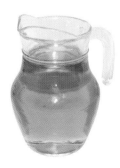

healthy growth. However, vinegar rinses should NOT be used on over-processed and chemically damaged hair, as it can be drying to very porous hair.

BASIC CIDER VINEGAR RINSE
Ingredients:
500ml water
200ml cider vinegar

Directions
1. Mix the vinegar and water together. You can experiment with the ratio: dry and coloured hair needs less vinegar, while oilier hair will benefit from a higher concentration.
2. After shampooing, tilt back your head and apply the vinegar rinse to your hair. Leave to sit for a couple of minutes. You can also add the mixture to a spray bottle and mist onto your hair whilst in the shower or bath.
3. Rinse the vinegar out of your hair with clean water. The smell of vinegar will dissipate once your hair dries.

CIDER VINEGAR RINSE FOR BLONDE HAIR
Chamomile is used to add shine while enhancing blond hues in the hair. It also promotes scalp health.

Ingredients:
200ml cider vinegar
500ml boiling water
2 chamomile tea bags or 3tbsp loose chamomile

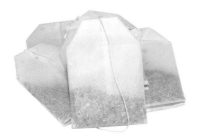

Do not put neat vinegar onto your hair as it can burn/aggravate the skin. Avoid contact with your eyes.

Directions
1. Add the tea bags to the boiling water. Cover and allow the mixture to cool and infuse for at least 20 minutes.
2. Strain the mixture if using loose chamomile. Mix in the cider vinegar.
3. After shampooing, pour the mixture over your hair. If you have long hair, dip the ends in a jug containing the mixture before pouring over the rest of the hair. Alternatively, apply to the hair using a spray bottle.
4. Leave on the hair for a couple of minutes then rinse with clean water.

CIDER VINEGAR RINSE FOR DARK HAIR
Rosemary stimulates hair growth and, when used as a rinse, will make hair gloriously glossy. Parsley moisturizes the hair, enriching colour and providing a nice lustre.

Ingredients:
200ml cider vinegar
500ml boiling water
1tbsp dried rosemary
1tbsp dried parsley

Directions
1. Add the loose herbs to the boiling water. Cover and allow the mixture to cool and infuse for at least 20 minutes.
2. Strain the loose herbs from the mixture. Mix in the cider vinegar.
3. After shampooing, pour the mixture over your hair. If you have long hair,

TIP

For an intense infusion of herbs, the cider vinegar recipes above can be made with fresh herbs and left to steep. Fill a large jar with a couple of handfuls of fresh herbs or nettles. Fill to the top with cider vinegar and leave to infuse for 2–3 weeks, shaking occasionally to release the oils from the herbs. Strain, dilute with water and use the rinse as described above.

dip the ends into a jug containing the mixture before pouring over the rest of the hair. Alternatively, apply to the hair using a spray bottle.
4. Leave on the hair for a couple of minutes then rinse with clean water.

CIDER VINEGAR RINSE FOR DANDRUFF
Cider vinegar and nettles have great cleansing and pH-balancing properties, which help to remove dandruff. Nettles are also rich in silica, which strengthens the hair and skin.

Ingredients:
200ml cider vinegar
500ml water
3tbsp dried nettles

Directions
1. Add the nettles to the boiling water. Cover and allow the mixture to cool and infuse for at least 20 minutes.
2. Strain the loose herbs from the mixture. Mix in the cider vinegar.
3. After shampooing, pour the mixture over your hair. If you have long hair, dip the ends into a jug containing the mixture before pouring over the rest of the hair. Alternatively, apply to the hair using a spray bottle.
4. Leave on the hair for a couple of minutes then rinse with clean water.

Dry Shampoo

Dry shampoo is perfect for removing excess oil and refreshing sets between washes.

FOR LIGHT HAIR
Ingredients:
4tbsp cornflower or arrowroot powder
3 drops of essential oil or lemon juice (optional)

Directions
Mix the powder and essential oil together. Use a large make-up brush to distribute into the roots or sprinkle directly onto the roots. Massage into the hair to absorb the excess oil and brush through to remove any excess powder. An old salt shaker makes a great applicator to dust the powder into the roots.

FOR DARK HAIR
Ingredients:
2tbsp cocoa powder
2tbsp cornflower or arrowroot powder
3 drops essential oil or lemon juice (optional)

Directions
Mix the powder and essential oil together. Use a large make-up brush to distribute into the roots or sprinkle directly onto the roots. Massage into the hair to absorb the excess oil and brush through to remove any excess powder. An old salt shaker makes a great applicator to dust the powder into the roots.

Spray Dry Shampoo

Ingredients:
1tbsp cornflower
4tbsp water
2tbsp rubbing alcohol
A few drops of essential oil or lemon juice (optional)
Spray bottle

Directions
Mix all the ingredients together in a bowl. Transfer to a spray bottle then lightly mist the mixture onto the roots of your hair and brush through. The hair will dry quickly as the alcohol evaporates. Shake the bottle before each use. Avoid using on dry or chemically damaged hair as the alcohol can be drying.

Cheesecloth Dry Shampoo

Wrap your brush in a piece of cheesecloth so that the bristles poke through the fabric. Brushing through the hair will naturally remove excess oil and dirt.

Pomades

Pomade is perfect for smoothing flyaway hairs and adding shine and hold to the hair whilst styling and brushing out. Castor oil is full of the vital nutrients, minerals and proteins required for healthy hair, such as vitamin E. It also has antibacterial properties.

Ingredients:
225g beeswax
1tbsp castor oil
1tbsp arrowroot powder
A few drops of essential oil

SUGGESTED OILS

Lemon and Tea Tree – with astringent properties, this is good for balancing oily hair.

Peppermint and Rosemary – stimulates circulation to the scalp, promoting healthy hair growth.

Chamomile and Lavender – perfect for dry hair

Nettle and Sage – help combat dandruff

If you prefer a very glossy-look pomade, omit the arrowroot.

Directions
Gently heat the beeswax in a double boiler and stir until the pellets dissolve. Next, add the castor oil and stir in the arrowroot, finishing with a few drops of essential oil. Pour in containers and leave to cool and solidify.

To use, take a pea-sized amount of pomade. At first, it will be hard but will soften as you work it between your fingers. Rub the pomade over your hands and style your hair as normal, being careful to avoid the roots, especially if you have fine hair. Do not overload your hair with the product; more can be added if required.

Creams and Masks

Honey Face Mask

Honey is naturally antibacterial. During the Second World War, it was used to help heal wounds as it stimulates skin growth and reduces inflammation and scarring. Therefore, honey makes a great face mask that heals skin breakouts and smoothes, nourishes and moisturizes the skin.

Apply a thin layer of honey to clean, dry skin. Leave on the skin for at least 10 minutes. Wash off with warm water and

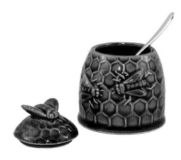

a flannel or piece of muslin. If the honey is very dense you can loosen it up with a few drops of warm water before applying.

Nourishing Eyelash Cream

Castor oil is very high in fatty acids and has many healing properties. For centuries it has been used externally and internally for numerous ailments, such as digestive problems, skin disorders and lacerations. The oil is great for growing long, healthy lashes, as the essential fatty acids boost blood circulation to the follicles, stimulating hair growth.

Ingredients:
    tsp cold pressed/cold processed
        castor oil
    1 tsp Vaseline

Directions
Mix the oil and Vaseline together and store in a small jar. Massage into the lashes at night after removing your make-up. Avoid getting the mixture in your eyes. Alternatively, apply the castor oil directly to your lashes with a clean mascara wand.

Cold Cream

Beeswax is used to help soften and firm the skin, while vitamin E cleanses and moisturizes. Vitamin E also has

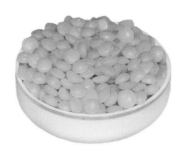

antioxidant properties that prevent skin from ageing. Almond and olive oils have a wide range of benefits for the skin, such as nourishing and plumping. Vitamin E is also a natural preservative, so your cream stays fresh. See below for a variety of different ways to use cold cream.

Ingredients:
    50ml almond oil
    50ml olive oil
    7g beeswax
    30ml rose water
    2 drops of chosen essential oil
    1 tsp vitamin E

Directions
Melt the beeswax pellets in a double boiler and stir until they dissolve. While still on the heat add the almond oil and olive oil, stirring well. Remove from the heat and pour into a glass or metal bowl and add the rose water, essential oil and vitamin E, whisking together briskly as the mixture cools. It should be the texture of thick, whipped cream. Spoon the mixture into a container and let it cool fully before use.

CLEANSER
Apply a generous amount of cold cream to your face and massage it into the skin. Wipe off the cream with a muslin, flannel or cotton wool (you can use a wet flannel or muslin if you prefer). Rinse your face thoroughly with warm water and pat dry.

FACE MASK
Cleanse your face with the cold cream. Apply a thin layer of the cream to your face and leave it to absorb for up to 10 minutes. Remove the cream with a muslin, flannel or cotton wool. Rinse your face with warm water and pat dry.

EYE MAKE-UP REMOVER
Scoop a small amount of the cold cream and massage it over your closed eyes in a circular motion. Use a muslin or cotton ball to wipe off the cream and any make-up residue.

BODY LOTION
Rub the cream into dry areas, such as elbows, for a moisture boost.

SHAVING CREAM
Use with a razor in place of shaving soap or gel.

CUTICLE AND HAND CREAM
Rub into the hands and cuticles for nourishment and a moisture boost.

Appendix: Pin Curl Diagrams

Shown below are the complete pin-curl setting patterns needed to re-create all of the step-by-step looks in the 'Classic Up Styles' and 'Classic Down Styles' chapters. If you wish to avoid heat and go down the more traditional route of wet setting this method is perfect for

you. Wet setting is also very useful for hair that is stubborn to curl, fragile hair or hair with chemical damage that needs to be protected from repeated heat styling.

For detailed information on the pin curl setting techniques needed to re-

create these diagrams, see the 'Creating Curls and Rolls' chapter and also make sure you read the 'Brushing out' chapter for tips and tricks of how to get the perfect finish when dressing out your set.

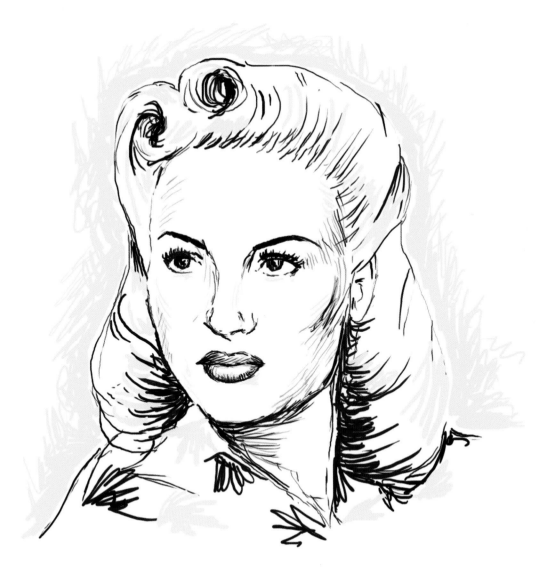

The Pin-Up

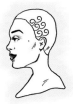

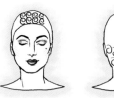

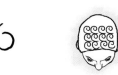

The Pin-Up set is created using half stem pin curls. Set the sides of the head with pin curls rolling upwards towards the face. The pin curls on the top and back of the head are set in rows with all pin curls rolling in the same direction.

The Carmen

 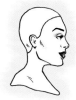

 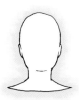

The Carmen: set the front section of the head in elevated pin curls.

The Rosie

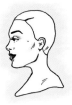 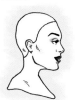

The Rosie: set the front section of the head in elevated pin curls rolling towards the face.

Charm School

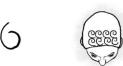

Charm School uses half stem pin curls. Set the sides in pin curls rolling under, away from the face. The top of the head is set with pin curls rolling in the same direction towards the side of the head. The back of the head is set in a skip wave.

The Classic Snood

 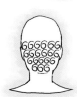

This set uses half stem pin curls. Set the top and sides of the head in large rows of pin curls, all rolling up and away from the face. The back is set in smaller pin curls all rolling in the same direction.

In the Navy

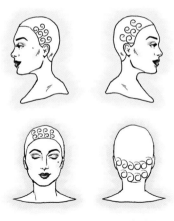

In the Navy: this set uses half stem pin curls. Set the top and sides of the head in medium to large pin curls, all rolling up and away from the face. The back is set in rows of pin curls all rolling in the same direction.

The Gibson Roll

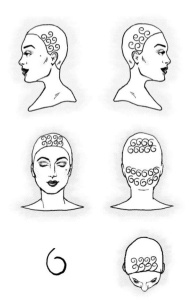

The Gibson Roll uses half stem pin curls. Set the top and sides of the head in large pin curls, all rolling up and away from the face. Set two rows of small to medium pin curls on the crown of the head. The lower back of the head is set in large pin curls all rolling in the same direction.

Forces Sweetheart

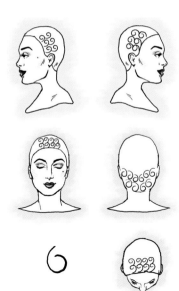

Forces Sweetheart: this set uses half stem pin curls. The top and sides of the head are set in large pin curls rolling up and away from the face. The back right of the head is set in large counterclockwise curls whilst the back left is set in clockwise curls.

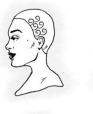
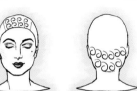
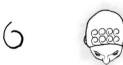

The Sophisticate

This set uses half stem pin curls. The top and the sides are set in large pin curls rolling up and away from the face. The back is set in large pin curls all rolling in the same direction.

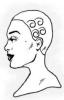

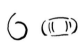
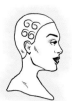
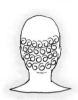

Lovely Lucille

This style uses half stem pin curls and elevated pin curls. Set the sides in large to medium pin curls, rolling under and away from the face. The top section is set in elevated pin curls rolling towards the face, while the back is set in small pin curls in a skip wave.

Origami

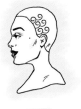

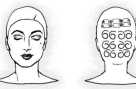

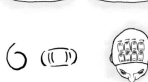

Origami: this style uses half stem pin curls and elevated pin curls. Set the sides in large pin curls rolling up and away from the face. The top section is set in elevated pin curls rolling towards the side of the head. The top back section of the head is set in elevated pin curl rolling downwards. The bottom right-hand side of the head is set in large clockwise pin curls, while the bottom left-hand side of the head is set in large counterclockwise pin curls.

The Chignon Style

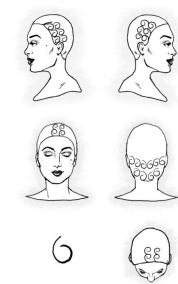

The Chignon Style uses half stem pin curls. Set the sides in large pin curls rolling away and downwards from the face. The top section is set with pin curls rolling downwards from the parting towards the side of the face. The back right of the head is set in large clockwise pin curls whilst the back left of the head is set in large,

Short and Sweet

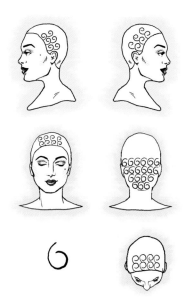

Short and Sweet: this style uses half stem pin curls. Set the top and sides of the head in pin curls rolling up and away from the face. The back is set in small to medium pin curls, all rolling in the same direction.

Hat Style

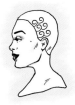 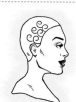

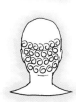

Hat Style uses half stem pin curls. Set the sides of the head in large pin curls rolling up and away from the face. Set the front right of the head in large counterclockwise curls and the top right in large clockwise curls.

The Smoothie

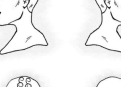

 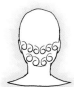

The Smoothie uses half stem pin curls. Set the sides of the head in large pin curls rolling under and away from the face. The top is set in large pin curls rolling downwards, away from the parting. Set the back also in large pin curls, with the back right in counterclockwise curls and the back left in clockwise curls.

Appendix: Pin Curl Diagrams

Half and Half

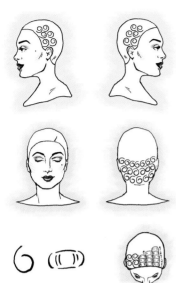

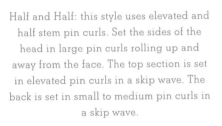

Half and Half: this style uses elevated and half stem pin curls. Set the sides of the head in large pin curls rolling up and away from the face. The top section is set in elevated pin curls in a skip wave. The back is set in small to medium pin curls in a skip wave.

The Crown

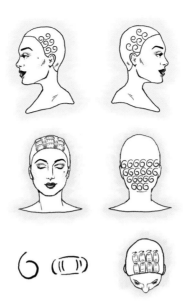

The Crown uses elevated and half stem pin curls. Set the sides of the head in large pin curls, rolling up and away from the face. The top is set rolling towards the side of the head in large elevated pin curls. The back is set in small to medium pin curls all rolling down in the same direction.

Old Hollywood

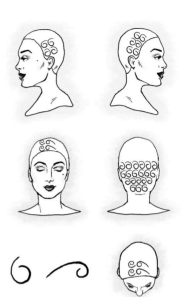

Old Hollywood: this style uses half stem and full stem pin curls. Set the sides of the head in medium to large pin curls rolling under and away from the face. The pin curls on the top of the head roll down and away from the parting, with the row closest to the parting being set in full stem pin curls. Set the back in medium to large pin curls set in a skip wave.

Sweeping Pompadour

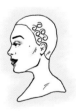 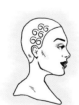

 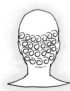

This style uses elevated and half stem pin curls. Set the sides in medium pin curls rolling under and away from the face. The top of the head is divided in to three sections. The middle section is set in medium, elevated pin curl rolling towards the face, while the right- and left-hand side sections are set in small elevated pin curls rolling towards the face. Set the back in small to medium pin curls all rolling downwards in the same direction.

The Bad Girl

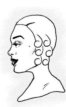

 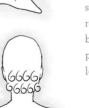

This style features a shadow wave and large stem pin curls. Make a wide side parting and comb in a shadow wave. Set the remaining ends and back of the hair in to pin curls with very long stems.

Cocktail Lounge

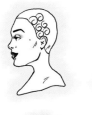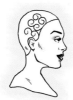
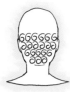
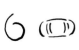

The Cocktail Lounge uses half stem and elevated pin curls. Set the sides of the head in medium to small pin curls rolling away from the parting in a skip wave. Set the back of the head in small to medium pin curls in a skip wave. The top of the head is set in small to medium elevated pin curls rolling towards the face.

The Lamarr

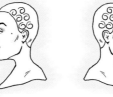

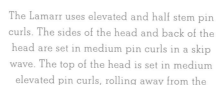

The Lamarr uses elevated and half stem pin curls. The sides of the head and back of the head are set in medium pin curls in a skip wave. The top of the head is set in medium elevated pin curls, rolling away from the

The Pageboy

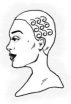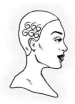
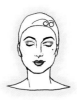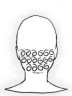

The Pageboy uses half and full stem pin curls. Set the sides of the head in small to medium pin curls, rolling under towards the face. Set the back right of the head in small to medium clockwise pin curls and the left in counterclockwise pin curls. The top of the head is set in small to medium half stem pin curls rolling towards the face in the same direction with the row closest to the parting being set in large stem pin curls.

The Perfect Pomp

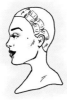
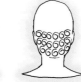
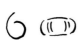

The Perfect Pomp uses elevated and half stem pin curls. Set the top and sides of the head in large elevated pin curls rolling away from the face. The back is set in small to medium pin curls all rolling in the same direction.

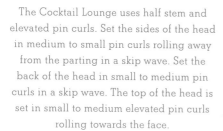

The Pompadour Wave

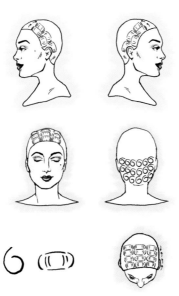

The Pompadour Wave uses elevated and half stem pin curls. Set the sides of the head in large elevated pin curls rolling away from the face. Set the top of the head in four rows of elevated pin curls. The three rows closest to the hairline are set in curls rolling away from the face, while the row closest to the crown is set rolling towards the face in the opposite direction. The back is set in small to medium pin curls all rolling in the same direction.

The Bombshell

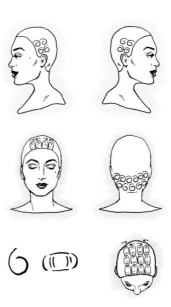

The Bombshell uses elevated and half stem pin curls. Set the sides of the head in small to medium pin curls in a skip wave. Set the top of the head in elevated pin curls rolling towards the side of the head in a skip wave. The back is set in small to medium pin curls in a skip wave.

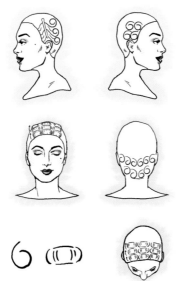

Glamour Girl

This style features a ridge wave, elevated pin curls and half stem pin curls. Set one side of the head in a ridge wave, forming the free ends of the hair in to half stem pin curls. Set the opposite side of the head in medium pin curls rolling towards the face, all in the same direction. The top of the head is set in elevated pin curls rolling away from the face. Set the back right-hand side of the head in clockwise curls and the left-hand side of the head in counterclockwise curls.

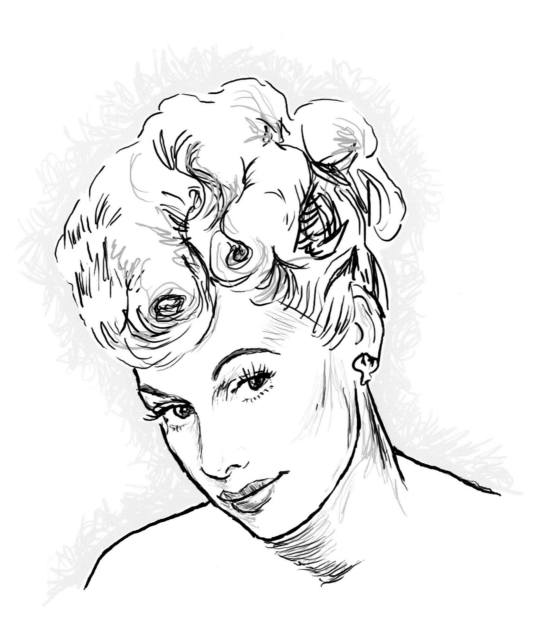

References

Chapter 1

1 Caroline Cox and Lee Widdows, Hair and Fashion, London, V&A Publications, 2005 (p. 64)
2 Richard Corson, Fashions in Hair: The First Five Thousand Years, London, Peter Owen Publishers, 2005 (p. 623)
3 Modern Shop Beauty Magazine, 1942
4 ibid.
5 Victory Hairpin Kit, Smith Victory Corporation, Buffalo, New York
6 Cox and Widdows, 2005 (p. 114)
7 Corson, 2005 (p. 622)

Chapter 2

8 May Smith, These Wonderful Rumours! A Young Schoolteacher's Wartime Diaries 1939–1945, London, Hachette Digital, 2012
9 Corson, 2005 (p. 658)

Chapter 3

10 Ern and Bud Westmore Beauty, Glamor and Personality, USA 2011 (p. 95)

Chapter 8

11 Westmore & Westmore, 2011 (p. 49)
12 ibid.
13 The Prelinger Archives, 1940s Make Up Video
15 ibid.

Acknowledgements

The author and publishers would like to thank the following for their help in producing this book.

Models

Rebecca Scott, Alex Outhwaite, Snow Daye, Anna Bailey, Sukhy Thandi, Lucy Armitage, Little Gem, Kiki DeVille, Miss Bamboo, Linda Owens, Patricia Lopes, Rachel Palmer, Stacey Stitch, Rebecca Mountfield-Pawlett, Constance Peach, Coco Lopes, Laura Norrey, Rebecca Forsythe, Laurie Lee, Heather Marie , Cat M Sleigh, Lori-Jade Barker, Natasha Harper, Linda Owens, Lizzie Garvey and Rebecca George.

Suppliers

Jewellery from Luxulite (http://luxulite.wix.com); outfits supplied by 20th Century Foxy (www.20thcenturyfoxy.com); illustrations from Becky Ryan Art (www.beckyryan.co.uk); nail tutorial and art by Five Finger Discount.

Photographers

Kim Nicholls from Madame Boudoir Photography Studio; Terry McNamara Photography (www.terrymcphotography.co.uk); Rachel Bywater Photography (www.rachelbywaterphotography.com);

Thank You

Many special people enabled to make this book possible. My wonderful family for supporting me throughout my career; thank you, Dad, David and Susie; Simon for patiently reading through my copy and helping my ideas make sense; my friends for always being there for me, with a special thank you to Lizzee for helping me with proof reading.
Thank you to the wonderful photographer Kim Nicholls for her skill in creating beautiful images – it is always wonderful to work with you; Terry McNamara for his stunning photos and ability to make shoots a fun place to be and Rachel Bywater for generally being amazing and her endless patience on perfecting the imagery for the book.
Thank you to Clare from 20th Century Foxy for supplying all of the outfits for the book – your authentic designs really capture the demure and glamorous feel of the 1940s.
Thank you to all the beautiful models – without your lovely faces the book would not have been possible.
Thank you to Becky Ryan for her artwork in the book. Becky would like to dedicate her illustrations for the book to her nana who sadly passed away before completion, and would have been very proud.

Index

Related Titles from Crowood

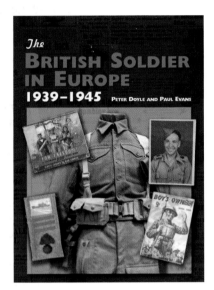

ISBN: 978 1 84797 102 9

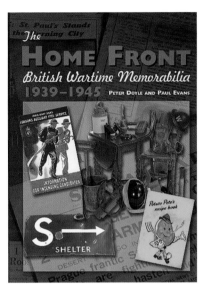

ISBN: 978 1 86126 927 0

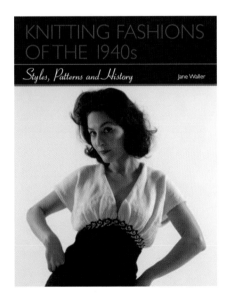

ISBN: 978 1 86126 862 4

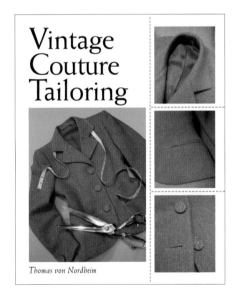

ISBN: 978 1 84797 373 3